Warning: This book is intended for people in good physical and psychological health who want to lose weight and tone up their abdominal muscles.

Before undertaking any dietary rebalancing and/or resuming any sporting activity, it is advisable to consult a doctor, particularly for people suffering from musculoskeletal disorders, digestive disorders, hormonal disorders or diabetes.

Anyone experiencing rapid weight gain should have a medical check-up to rule out any possible pathology.

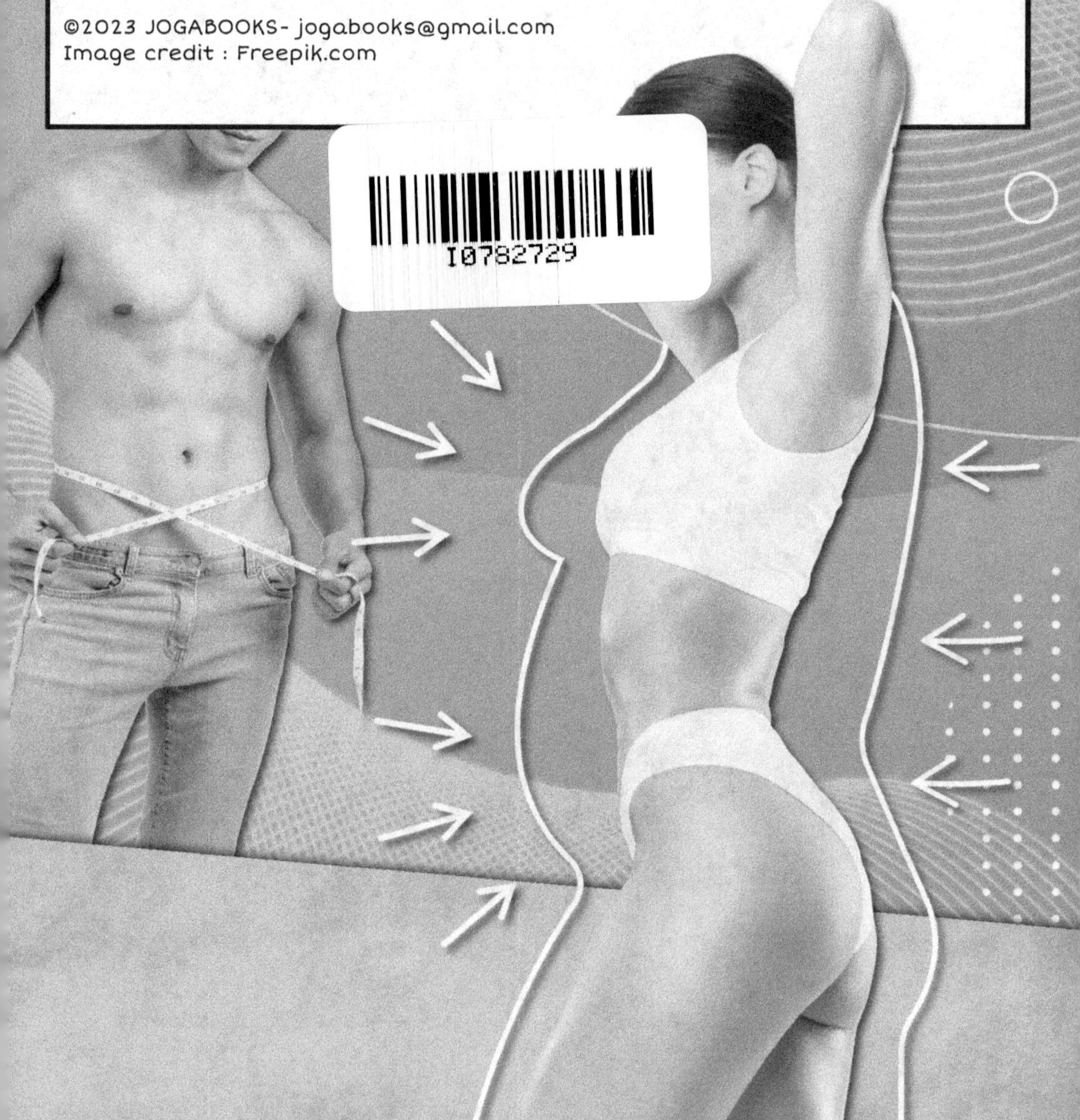

CONTENTS

Introduction ... 4

PART 1. What you need to know ... 6
What is a fat belly? ... 8
Fat ... 10
The risks of being overweight ... 14
Overweight myths ... 16
How to get a flat stomach? ... 18
Be motivated ... 20
Body mass index ... 23
Basal metabolic rate ... 24
Total energy expenditure ... 25

PART 2. Food ... 28
How to eat well? ... 30
Nutrients ... 32
Macronutrients ... 34
Micronutrients ... 38
Other elements ... 40
How to calculate calories ... 42
How to weigh food ... 47
Food quality ... 50
Caloric deficit ... 52
Macronutrient ratio ... 54
Important rules ... 58
What if I'm hungry? ... 60
Cheat meals ... 62

PART 3. Physical activity   64
Abdominal muscles   66
Back posture   68
How to tone stomach and back   72
Transverse   74
Obliques   76
Rectus abdominis   78
How to stretch the back   79
The back   80
Workout example   82
How to burn fat   84
List of sports activities   86
A healthy body   88
Hormonal system   89
Sleep   90
Stress   92
In conclusion   94

APPENDIX   96
Nutrition tables   98
Meat   99
Cold cut / charcuterie   100
Fish and seafood   101
Starchy foods   102
Vegetables   103
Dairy products   104
Desserts and cakes   105
Fruits   106
Drinks   107
Other foods   108
Calorie intake per day   109

INTRODUCTION

Many of us dream of a flat stomach.

We all want to be able to go to the beach or the pool without complexes, to look at ourselves in the mirror with pride, or simply to be able to wear those jeans (or that dress) that looked so good on us a few years ago. At one time or another, we've probably felt embarrassed by the way others look at us.

It's not just a question of aesthetics.

Our complexes have a major impact on our self-esteem and self-confidence, and the repercussions are felt in our daily lives.

Our health is also affected, and the risks associated with being overweight are not to be overlooked.

Perhaps we've already tried to lose a little weight, with disappointing results. Is this inevitable? Of course not!

Let's imagine for a moment that we've achieved our goal. Let's imagine that every morning, we wake up feeling light - both physically and emotionally. Imagine walking down the street with confidence and self-assurance. Wouldn't that be great?

In reality, and this is good news, it's not that complicated to get a flat stomach.
It requires a few adjustments, a little action, a nice dose of motivation, and perseverance, but it's probably less of a sacrifice than we might imagine.

Throughout this book, we'll take you step-by-step through everything you need to know and do to reach your goal.

And let's be clear from the outset: this is not about imposing a strict diet of frustration and deprivation, which would be doomed to failure.
On the contrary, we want everyone to become autonomous, by adjusting each step, each piece of advice, to their lifestyle and daily imperatives.

Lao-tzu said, "If you give a man a fish, he will eat for a day. If you teach him to fish, he will eat for a lifetime."

When we close this book, we'll know why our bellies aren't as flat as we'd like, and we'll understand why we have a few misplaced curves.
Whether we're male or female, 20 or 50, we'll be able to reach our goal and adopt a healthier lifestyle.

Let's get ready to embark on this journey together, to free our bodies from complexes and improve our well-being.

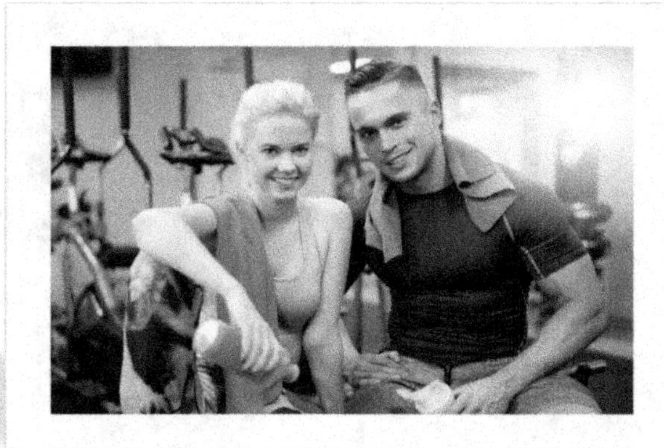

Emilie & Sacha

WHAT YOU NEED TO KNOW

What is a big belly? What is fat and how does it form? What are the risks of being overweight? How do I calculate my BMI?

In this first part, we're going to broaden our knowledge and take stock of our initial situation.

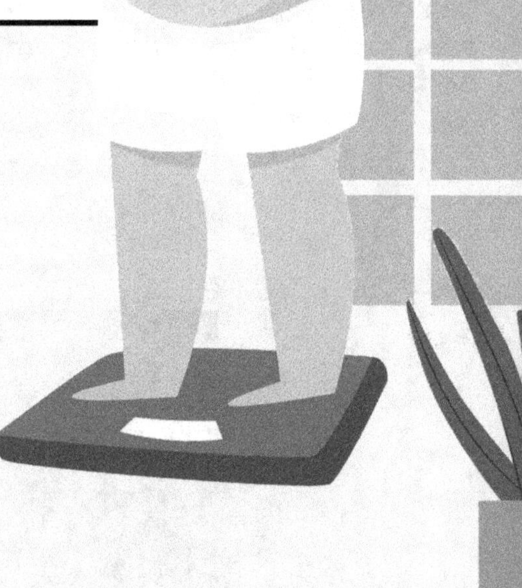

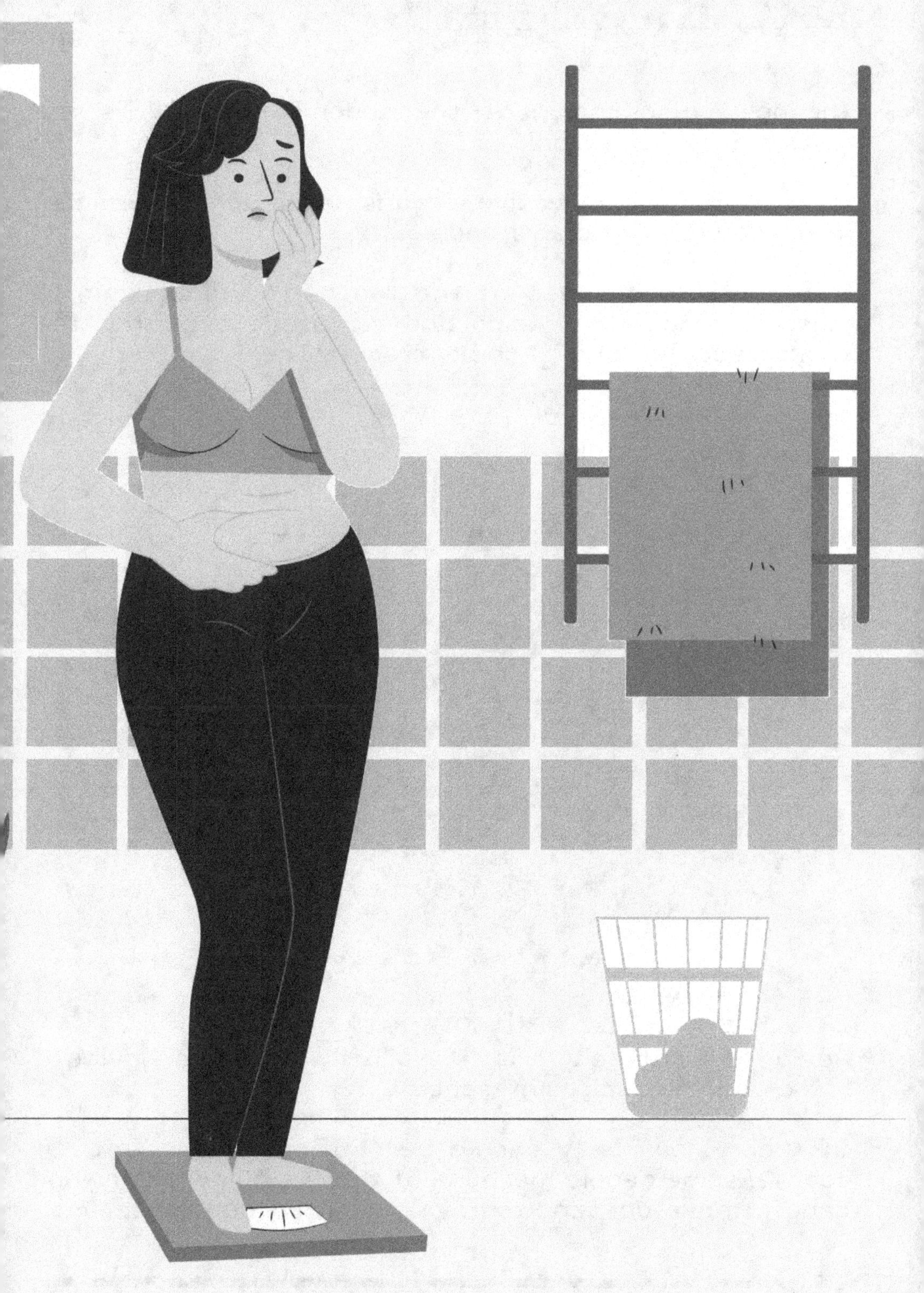

WHAT IS A FAT BELLY?

The belly, also known as the abdominal cavity, is the lower part of the trunk.

It contains the digestive organs (stomach, intestines, liver, pancreas), kidneys and spleen.

This cavity is bounded at the top by the diaphragm (a musculo-tendinous membrane located beneath the thoracic cavity) and at the bottom by the pelvis.

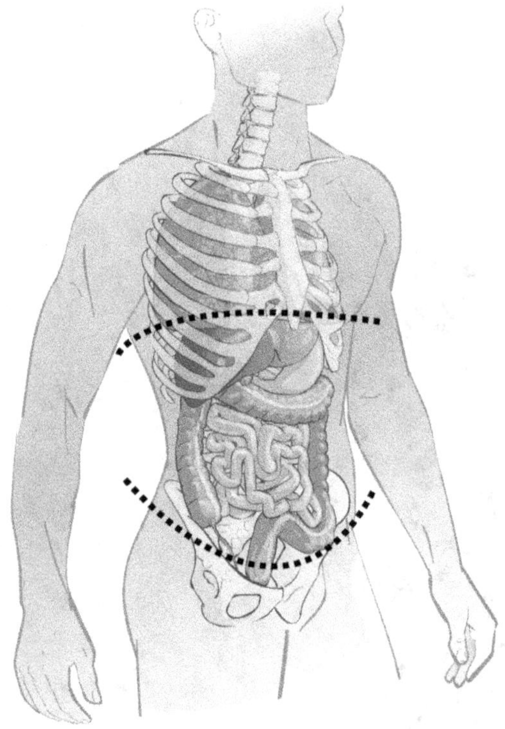

Do I have a fat belly or not?

Having a " fat belly " (or " big belly ") means having a large abdominal circumference.

In theory, our belly should be flat or almost flat. Of course, some people, because of their age, morphology or genetic make-up, tend to have a slightly rounded belly.

There are medical standards and measurements to define "big belly" or abdominal distension.

However, these measures do not take into account one fundamental aspect: Us!

How do we feel when we look at our belly? Do we like it?

If this book is in our hands, it's almost certainly because we're not totally at ease with our bodies.

Perhaps we're influenced by society's aesthetic standards. Perhaps we simply want to look good. Perhaps it's a question of health.

Whatever the reason. What's important is our willingness to change. If we think our belly is too rounded, let's do something about it.

Most often, an increase in volume in the abdominal cavity is caused by an accumulation of fat mass, but there are also other factors, such as slackening of the abdominal muscles and poor posture (pelvis and back).

Accumulation of several of these factors is not uncommon. Overweight people (even those who are slightly overweight) often experience varying degrees of muscle relaxation in their abdominal muscles, which in turn can lead to postural problems.

Finally, our lifestyles (stress, lack of sleep...) can lead to hormonal disturbances that accentuate weight gain.

Let's take a closer look at factor No. I: FAT !

FAT

Fat, also known as adipose tissue or fat mass, is an important element in the proper functioning of our bodies, and plays a number of roles.

Energy storage: Fat is an energy reserve. In simple terms, when the body needs energy, a hormonal signal releases certain fat cells (triglycerides), which are then broken down into glycerol and fatty acids. These, in turn, are released into the bloodstream and transported to tissues (such as muscles) for use as fuel. It is estimated that 100 grams (3.5 Oz) of fat mass can produce around 750 Kcal.

Thermal insulation: Fat acts as a thermal insulator, enabling the body to better regulate its internal temperature and better resist variations in external temperatures.

Organ protection: Fat surrounding certain organs (heart, kidneys, liver) provides protection in the event of shock.

Hormonal regulation: Certain fat cells are involved in the production of hormones such as cortisol, testosterone, estrogen and progesterone.

The three types of fat

White fat: This is the most common form of fat in our bodies. It is mainly subcutaneous (under the skin) and distributed throughout the body, in varying quantities. Generally, and especially in cases of excess, it is found mainly on the abdomen, hips, thighs, buttocks and lower back.

White fat is primarily used for energy storage and hormone production.

Brown fat: Much less prevalent than white fat, brown fat is found mainly in the neck and shoulders. Its role is essentially thermal.

This type of fat is more prevalent in infants.

Beige fat: There's another type of adipose tissue, called beige fat.

Discovered recently, this fat is the result of the transformation of white fat under the effect of external stimuli, notably exposure to cold. Beige fat has properties similar to those of brown fat, and is therefore involved in thermal regulation.

Body fat percentage

Normal body fat (i.e. the percentage of adipose tissue present in the body) varies mainly according to sex and age.

For men, normal body fat is between 10 and 25%.

For women, normal body fat is between 20 and 35%.

Body fat levels are naturally higher in women. This is due in particular to the greater need for hormonal regulation (for menstrual cycles, for example), as well as to compensate for possible needs during pregnancy.

A body fat percentage between 25 and 30% for men and between 35 and 40% for women is an indicator of overweight.

A body fat percentage in excess of 30% for men and 40% for women is an indicator of obesity.

Belly fat

Abdominal fat is unique in that it can be found both under the skin (subcutaneous fat) and in the abdominal cavity (visceral fat).

Subcutaneous fat is easy to identify. Simply pinch the skin of the abdomen to feel the fatty mass between the skin and the abdominal muscles.

Visceral fat is more difficult to estimate. Only medical imaging methods (MRI, for example) can provide accurate results.

However, a high waist circumference, particularly in relation to the hip circumference, is a sign to be taken into account. Generally speaking, a very rounded belly indicates a high visceral fat mass.

Impedance-meter scales, which are still affordable, give relatively accurate results.

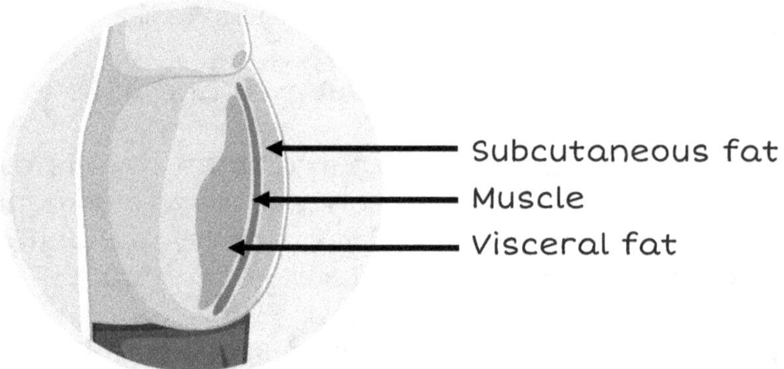

How does fat form?

Fat is formed when there is an imbalance between energy intake and energy expenditure.

To measure energy intake and expenditure, we use a unit of energy measurement called Kilocalorie (Kcal).

Energy intake comes from everything we eat and drink. Each food has a different energy intake (or caloric intake). For example, 100 grams (3.5 Oz) of French fries provide around 250 Kcal, but 100 grams (3.5 Oz) of raw carrot provide 40 Kcal.

Energy expenditure comes from the functioning of our body.
Our bodies are constantly expending energy, whether to breathe, walk, talk, watch TV, play sports or maintain body heat. This expenditure depends on the activity performed. For example, an hour's walk on flat ground expends an average of 150 Kcal, but an hour's cycling at a speed of 30 km/h (18.6 mph) expends between 600 and 1000 Kcal.

When energy intake exceeds energy expenditure, the body stores the excess calories as fat.

However, this excess must be regular, relatively large and occur over a relatively long period.

If the energy surplus does not occur regularly, or if it is small, the increase in fat mass will be virtually nil. Some people tend to store fat more easily than others, and conversely, some people store little fat mass even when they have a large caloric surplus.

Our genetic make-up plays an important role in these differences, but it's not the only cause.

Our metabolism (i.e. all chemical and biological transformations within our body) also plays an important role, and this is where hormonal functioning comes into play.

Finally, the composition of our diet plays a very important role. Some foods are much more conducive to fat storage than others.

THE RISKS OF BEING OVERWEIGHT

Although fat is essential for our bodies to function properly, too much of it can lead to significant problems.

Indeed, overweight and obesity present significant health risks. Of course, these risks are related to the extent of overweight and to genetic factors.

Cardiovascular disease
Being overweight is a major contributor to the development of cardiovascular disease (high blood pressure, cardiac arrhythmia, risk of heart attack, etc.).

Type 2 diabetes
Being overweight significantly increases the risk of developing type 2 diabetes, which creates insulin resistance and therefore high blood sugar levels.

Cancer
Being overweight increases the risk of developing cancer, including breast, colon, esophageal, stomach, kidney, liver, pancreatic and uterine cancer.

Joint disorders
Excess weight, and the resulting pressure on the joints, leads to problems such as inflammation, joint pain and osteoarthritis.

Respiratory problems
Excess weight can lead to respiratory problems, including sleep apnea.

Liver risks

Being overweight can increase the risk of liver disease, particularly steatosis (accumulation of fat in the liver).

Psychological impact

In addition to its impact on physical health, being overweight often has consequences for mental health. These risks, all too often underestimated, must be taken seriously.

Being overweight, even when it's only a little, can lead to a reduction in self-esteem and self-confidence.

In some cases, this can lead to exclusion, stigmatization and discrimination.

These situations can lead, among other things, to depression and relational difficulties, with repercussions for both personal and professional life.

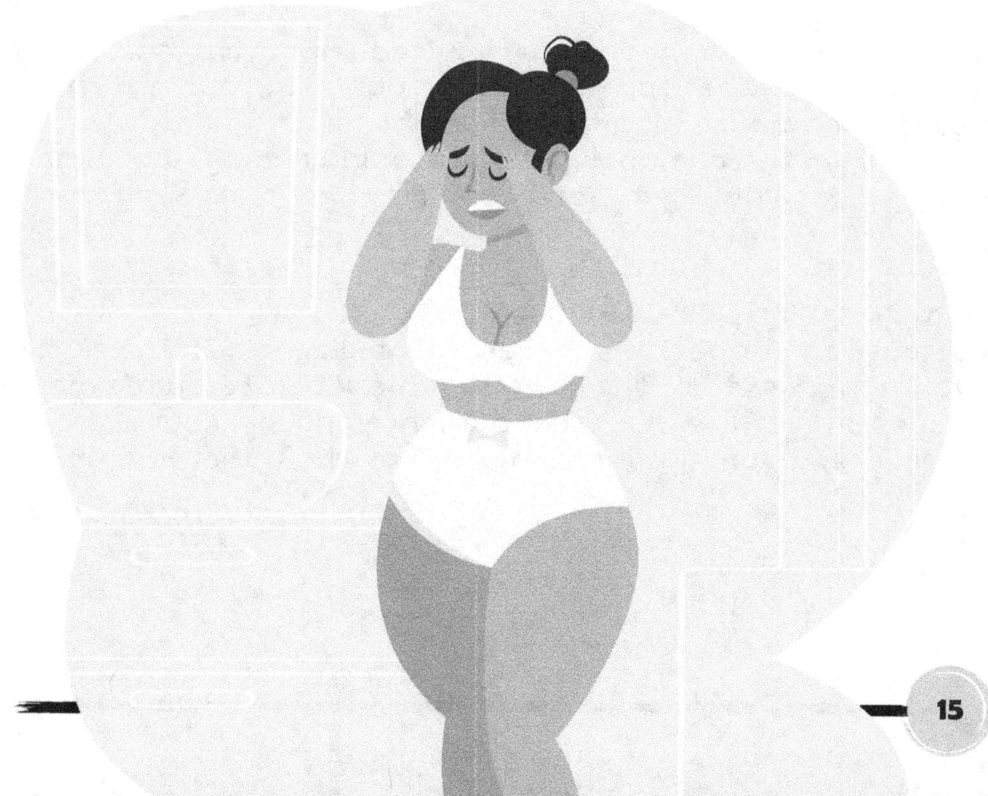

OVERWEIGHT MYTHS

There are many myths about being overweight, and it's important to clear them up right away.

Restrictive diets

As we'll see in this book, it's important to restrict certain foods in order to eliminate body fat. However, overly restrictive diets, while they may result in temporary weight loss, are totally ineffective in the long term. Recent studies have shown that 95% of dieters regained weight (sometimes even more than before the diet) within a few months.

You should also beware of certain diets that restrict or favor a particular family of foods. These diets can lead to deficiencies which can have a detrimental impact on the body's ability to burn fat.

Slimming creams

Slimming creams have very limited effectiveness. They may improve the appearance of our skin, but they can never bring about significant weight loss.
 Beware of the composition of certain creams, which can have undesirable side-effects, such as skin irritation.

Appetite suppressant pills

Not only are appetite suppressant pills less effective (or even non-existent), they are often associated with more or less harmful side effects (high blood pressure, mood disorders, insomnia, inflammation of the pancreas, etc.).

Sweat belts

The famous sweat belts, usually sold with the promise of targeted fat loss, actually have absolutely no effect whatsoever. As their name suggests, they make you sweat, and that's all. As sweat is made up of water and minerals, it's easy to see that a sweat belt will never melt fat.

Low-fat foods

Low-fat foods can sometimes be an interesting alternative to products that are too rich. Beware, however, of the composition of some of these foods, which may contain substances of industrial origin that can be harmful to health. Be sure to read labels carefully.

Targeting fat loss

Targeting fat loss is very difficult (if not impossible). So, for example, it's a myth that you can only lose belly fat. The same goes for thighs, buttocks, etc...
In reality, when the conditions are right for the body to reduce our fat mass, this loss will be generalized rather than localized.
That said, it's a very good thing, if only from an aesthetic point of view.

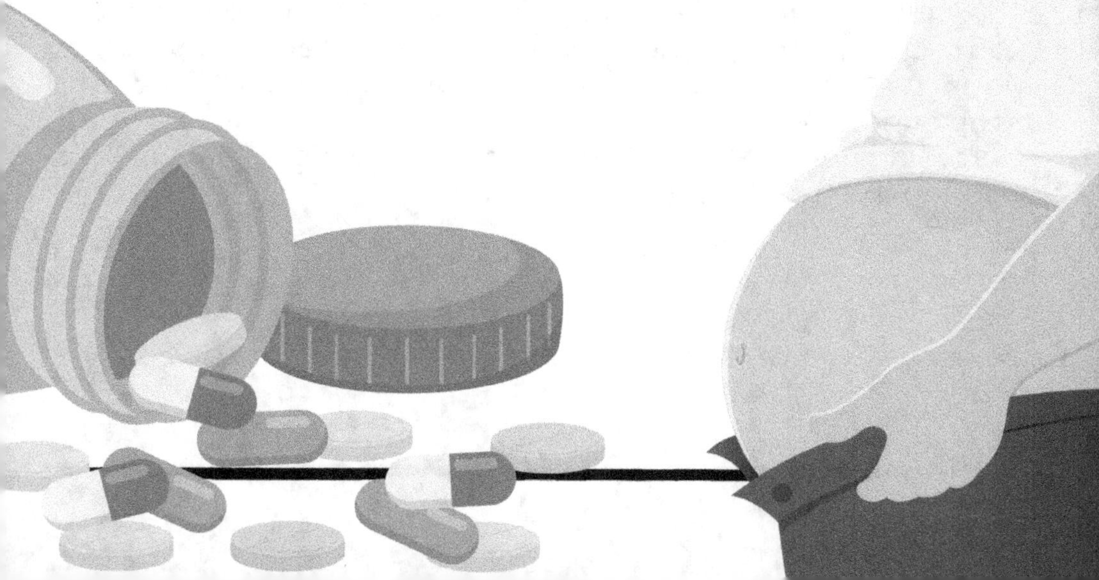

HOW TO GET A FLAT STOMACH?

As we've just seen, being overweight has a potentially harmful impact on our physical and psychological health, and there's no miracle product for losing weight.

If we want to lose belly fat, we need to tackle the most important factor: excess fat.
We also need to tighten our abdominal muscles and correct our posture, if necessary.

To do this, we first need to take action on our diet. Diet, as we shall see in the following pages, is the major cause of fat accumulation in our bodies.

Next, we'll take action on our physical activity, which conditions our energy expenditure (and therefore our ability to burn fat), but also our muscle tone and posture.

Finally, we'll look at various parameters, such as stress and sleep, to improve our hormonal functioning and promote our body's natural regulation.

The whole approach is progressive. There's no question of following a drastic diet, or going for a 2-hour run every day.

That would certainly be an effective method, but not one that can be sustained over the long term. And what happens afterwards, when we abandon our diet and stop running?
Quite simply, we'll gain back all the weight we've lost, and maybe even more.

If we want lasting results, we need to understand how our bodies work, and we need to change certain behaviors. That's how we'll reach our goal, and that's how we'll maintain our weight and keep our tummy flat.

Each step in this book can be adapted to suit your starting situation and your goals.

Whatever our age, whatever our sex, we'll be able to take concrete action to achieve a flat stomach.

After all, it's easy, isn't it?

All you need is a minimum of motivation!

Let's talk about that.

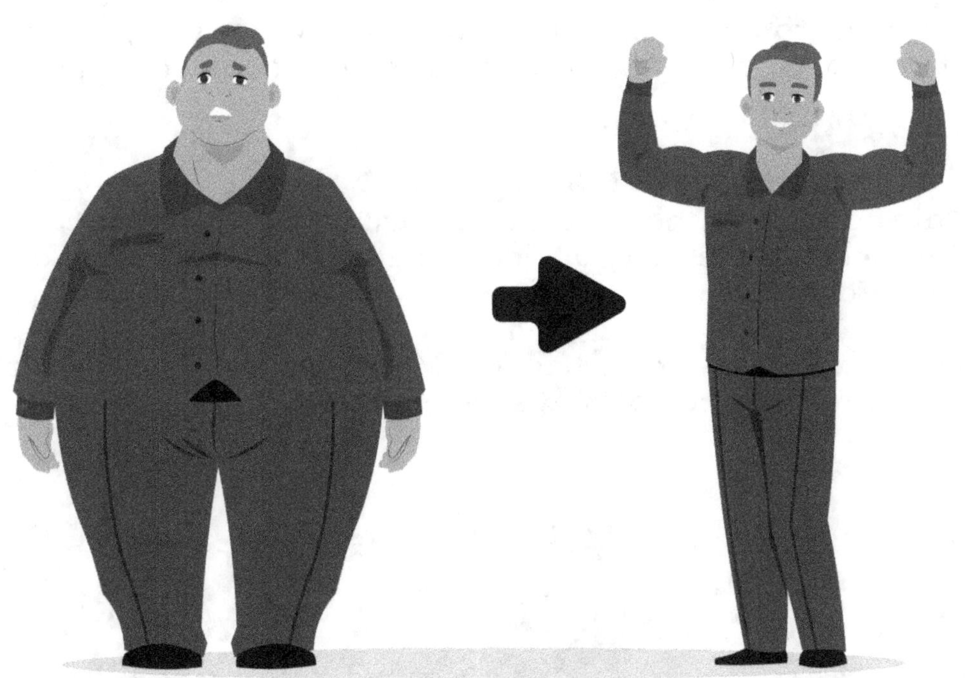

BE MOTIVATED

Motivation is our fuel. Without it, we won't find the energy we need to make any effort, be it dietary or physical.

Motivation is the key to your success.

Here are a few tips on how to stay motivated:

Set goals

Setting an objective means visualizing a result, a goal to be achieved. A goal must be realistic and time-bound.

For example, I want to lose 5 cm (2 inches) around my waist in 2 months, or I want to be able to wear that dress this summer, or quite simply, I want to feel good about my body in 6 months' time.

We need to visualize our goal regularly. Let's try to feel the positive changes that achieving our goal will bring.

Don't watch your weight too much

Gaining weight doesn't necessarily mean gaining body fat. Regular exercise will increase your muscle mass, and therefore your weight.

For example, it's best to measure your waist circumference to estimate your results.

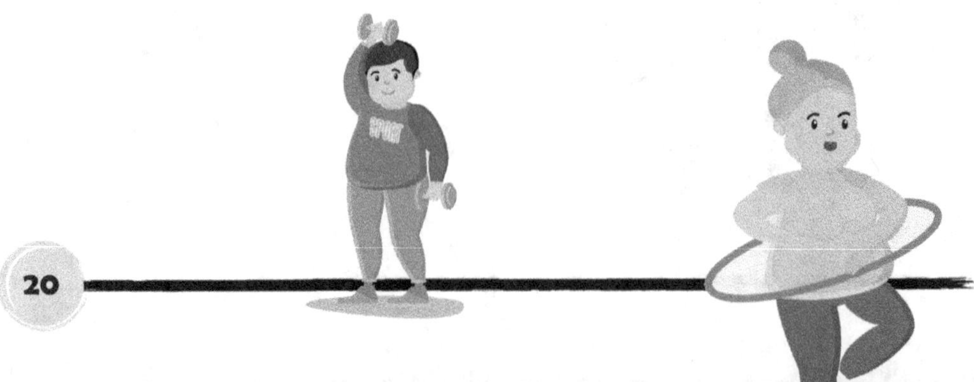

Taking your time

Setting too big a goal in too short a time is a very good way to fail.

Whether in terms of food or sport, you mustn't go from one extreme to the other.

No frustration

Rebalancing your diet sometimes requires effort and compromise. But be careful not to fall into constant frustration, which would be totally counterproductive.

Create new habits

Changing our habits can be complicated. Cooking a healthy meal instead of going out for fast food, getting active instead of watching TV from the comfort of the sofa...

Making a schedule can help us change our habits more easily.
Depending on our schedule, we can define our cooking times, our physical activity times, our bedtimes...

No excuses!

We were supposed to exercise for 30 minutes this evening, but we've had a tiring day? We were supposed to cook a healthy meal, but there's a really interesting program on TV? We'll always find an excuse to avoid the effort.

So, no excuses, and let's do what we have to do to reach our goal.

BMI, TMR AND TDEE

First of all, we'll need to make a few calculations to define our starting point and estimate our caloric requirements.

It's very important to carry out this step in order to have a baseline from which to adapt our diet and energy expenditure.

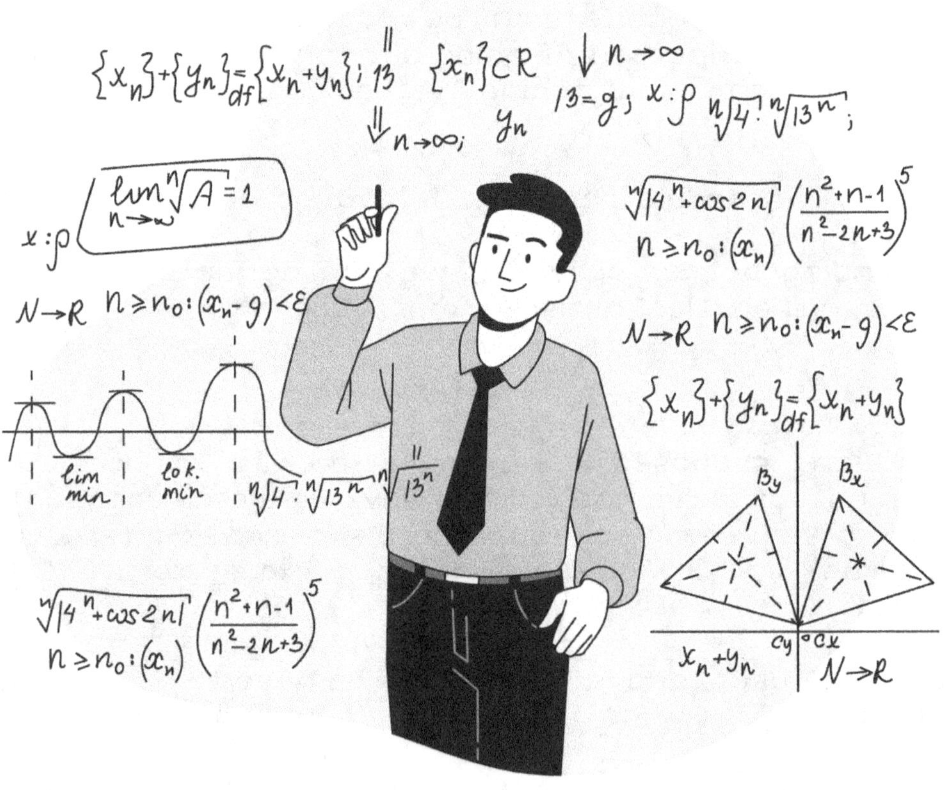

BODY MASS INDEX

The body mass index, or BMI, is a simple calculation used to assess a person's corpulence, based on two parameters: height and weight.

The calculation is as follows:
International units: WEIGHT (Kg) / (HEIGHT (m))^2
Imperial units: WEIGHT (Lb) / (SIZE (in))^2 X 703

Whatever the method of calculation, the results will be virtually identical.

Example with the metric system for a person measuring 1.70 m and weighing 80 kg:
80 ÷ (1.70)^2 = 80 ÷ 2.89 = 27.68
This person's BMI is 27.68.

Once the BMI has been calculated, compare it with the values below:
BMI under 18.5: Underweight
BMI between 18.5 and 24.9: Normal weight
BMI between 25 and 30: Overweight
BMI over 30: Obesity

To return to our example, this person is therefore overweight.

BMI gives an indication of overall body mass, and it's important to calculate it for estimation purposes.

Be careful, however, as BMI has its limitations: It doesn't differentiate between age or sex, and it can't distinguish fat mass from muscle or bone mass.
So an athletic person may have a high BMI, but not be overweight.

Calculate your BMI now!

BASAL METABOLIC RATE

The basic metabolic rate, or BMR, is the number of calories our body needs to perform vital functions (breathing, circulation, temperature regulation, etc.).

Unlike BMI, calculation methods take gender and age into account. There are several formulas, and all give a similar result. Most methods use the international system of units. So you'll need to convert your weight into KG and your height into CM.

Let's take the Mifflin St Jeor method:

For MEN :
(10 X weight in Kg) + (6.25 X height in cm) - (5 X age in years) + 5

For WOMEN :
(10 X weight in Kg) + (6.25 X height in cm) - (5 X age in years) - 161

The result will be an estimate of the number of Kcal our body needs ONLY to maintain vital functions over the course of a day (24 hours).

Let's take the example of a woman weighing 60 kg, measuring 1.60 m and aged 35.

BMR = (10 X 60) + (6.25 X 160) - (5 X 35) - 161
BMR = 600 + 1000 - 175 - 161
BMR = 1264

This woman therefore has a basic metabolic rate of 1264 Kcal.

Let's calculate our BMR!

TOTAL ENERGY EXPENDITURE

We're now going to calculate our total daily energy expenditure (TDEE).

Firstly, we need to apply a coefficient to our result (BMR) based on our energy expenditure, in order to estimate the total number of calories required over a day.

These coefficients are therefore directly linked to our level of daily physical activity.

They are mainly determined on the basis of overall physical activity (including physical activity resulting from professional activity) and sporting activity.

They are classified as follows :

Sedentary: Very little physical activity during the day, and no sporting activity.

Moderately active: little physical activity and/or low-intensity sports activities.

Active: Moderate physical and sporting activity.

Very active: Intense physical activity and/or sports activities.

Intensive: Very intense physical and/or sporting activity.

To determine which category we fall into, we need to take into account our physical activity as a whole.

For example, if we have an office job (sedentary), but we do an hour's boxing every evening, then we're in the "active" or "very active" category.

Which category are we in?

Once the category has been determined, we need to apply the coefficient to our BMR to obtain the value, in Kcal, of our total energy expenditure (also known as TDEE).

The coefficients are :
Sedentary: X 1.2
Moderately active: X 1.375
Active: X 1.55
Very active: X 1.725
Intensive: X 1.9

Let's go back to our example with the 35-year-old woman. Her BMR is 1264 Kcal.

She has an office job, and uses her car to get there. She practices yoga (a moderately intense sporting activity) 3 times a week for 1 hour.

We can therefore consider her to be in the "moderately active" category.

Let's take her BMR and apply the corresponding coefficient.

1264 X 1.375 = 1738

Her total daily energy expenditure (TDEE) is therefore 1738 Kcal.

Let's imagine that this woman pays a little attention to her diet and consumes, on average, 1750 Kcal per day.

As the difference between intake and expenditure is almost identical, this woman's weight will change very little, if at all, and very slowly.

Now, let's imagine that this woman's diet is too rich and she consumes 2000 Kcal per day.

Her energy intake far exceeds her energy expenditure (i.e. her needs). The body will store the excess energy and this woman's body fat will increase.

Finally, let's imagine that this woman watches her diet closely to lose weight, and consumes 1400 Kcal per day. Her energy intake is much lower than her energy expenditure (this is called a caloric deficit), and she will gradually lose body fat.

Estimating our energy needs is therefore an essential step if we want to reduce our body fat.

We've already calculated our BMR. Let's apply the coefficient corresponding to our situation to obtain our TDEE.

What are our energy requirements (TDEE)?

Now that we know what our energy needs are, we can start by taking action on our calorie intake, and therefore on our diet.

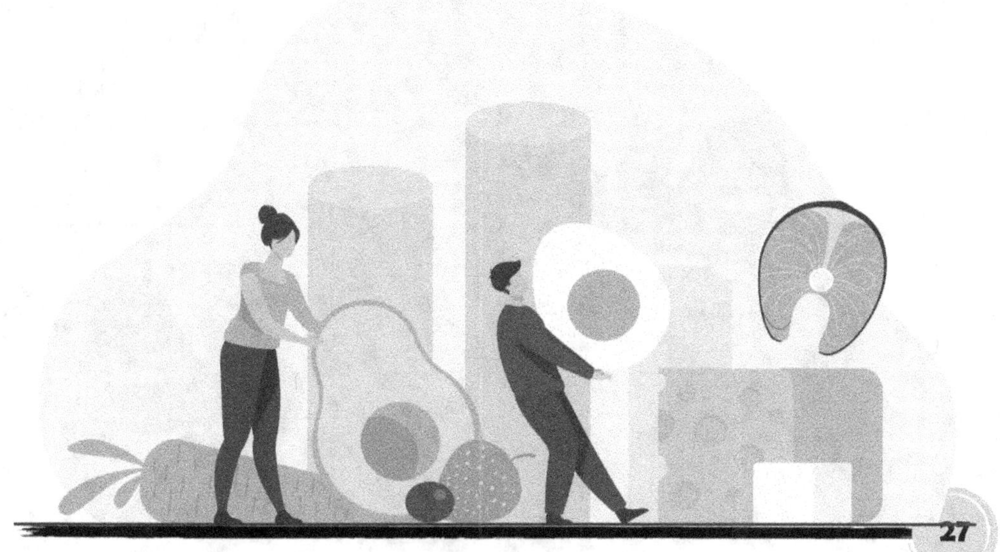

FOOD

What we eat has a major influence on our physical and mental well-being. Every food we eat has an impact on our health. What we eat is the primary cause of fat accumulation, in our bellies and elsewhere.

In this section, we'll take a look at the different nutrients and their roles, and see how we can adopt a healthy diet that meets our needs.

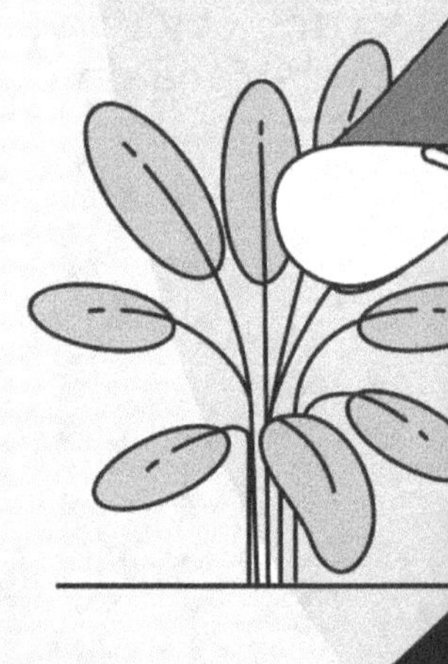

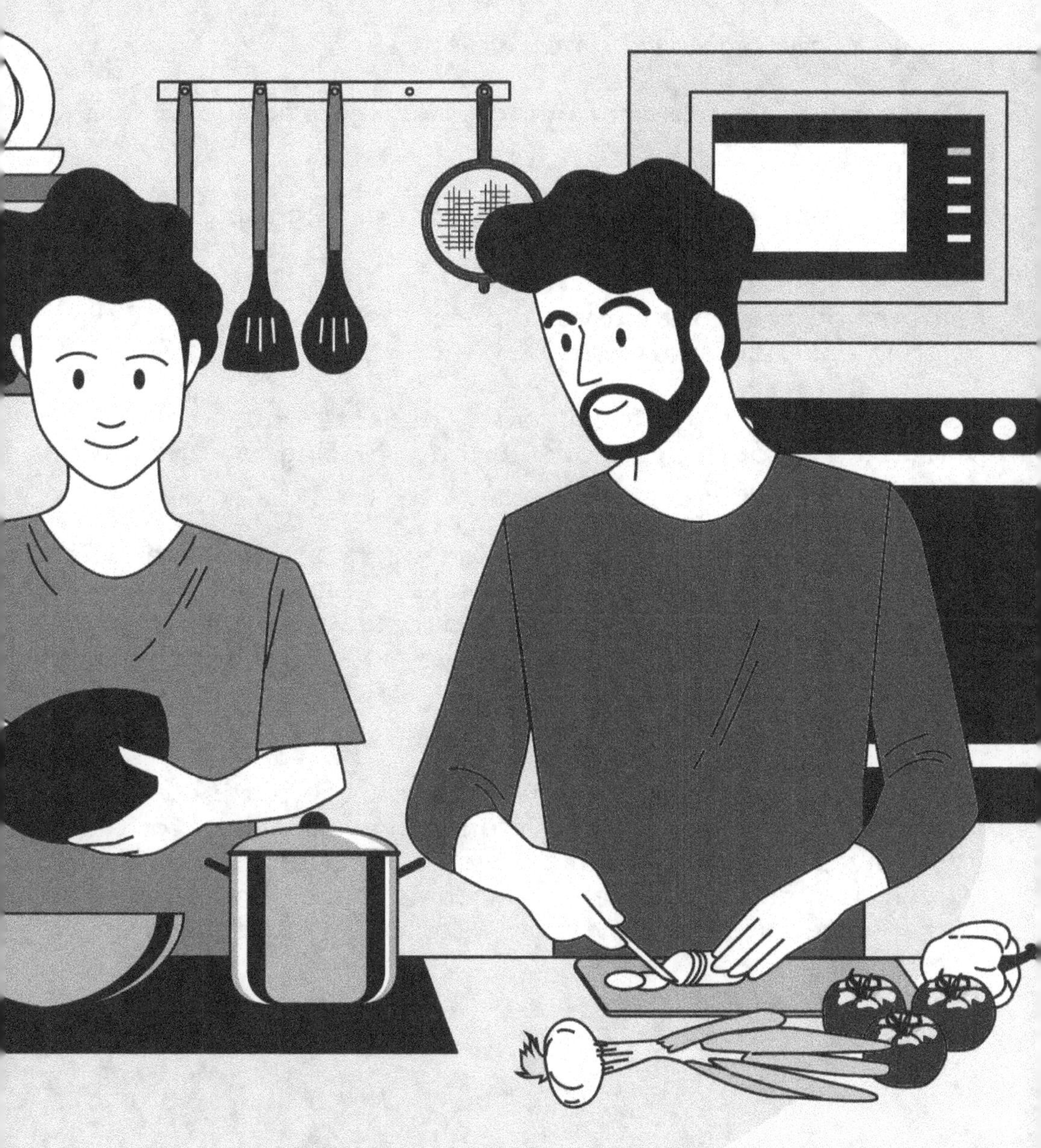

HOW TO EAT WELL ?

Good nutrition is the key to a flat stomach, avoiding excess weight and staying healthy.

So we need to control what we eat.

To do this, we need to act on two pillars: quantity and quality.

Controlling the quantitative aspect enables us to manage our calorie intake.

Mastering the qualitative aspect ensures a healthy diet, rich in essential nutrients.

Quantitative and qualitative aspects are therefore linked, and acting on one without acting on the other makes no sense.

Once again, it's not a question of drastically reducing the quantity of food swallowed. This would have a harmful psychological impact and would be doomed to failure in the long term. What's more, it's highly likely that such a diet would lead to deficiencies that would have repercussions on our health.

Nor is it a question of eliminating all the little pleasures of taste. It's important, from time to time, to treat ourselves to our favorite cake, or any other food that gives us pleasure. Under no circumstances should we fall into excessive deprivation. Eating should remain a pleasure.

Yes, it is possible to lose belly fat by eating chocolate, ice cream and hamburgers from time to time...

But let's face it, we're still going to have to make some changes to our diet.

These changes will achieve two goals:
* Create a caloric deficit, which will force our body to draw energy from fat mass.
* Improving our nutritional intake, which will improve our body's overall functioning and health.

To achieve these goals, we need a good understanding of nutrition.

So, to begin with, we're going to take a look at the nutrients in our food, and discover their role and impact on our bodies.

NUTRIENTS

A nutrient is an elementary component provided by food and assimilated by our body.

There are two main families of nutrients: Macronutrients and micronutrients.

Macronutrients

Macronutrients are nutrients that the body needs in large quantities. They provide the energy our bodies need to function properly, as well as certain essential components.

They are therefore the main components of our diet.

There are 3 groups of macronutrients: Proteins, carbohydrates and lipids.

Micronutrients

Micronutrients are also essential nutrients for our bodies, but in much smaller quantities.

Unlike the three different groups of macronutrients, micronutrients do not provide energy.

The main micronutrients are vitamins, minerals and trace elements. Other elements, such as probiotics, are also present.

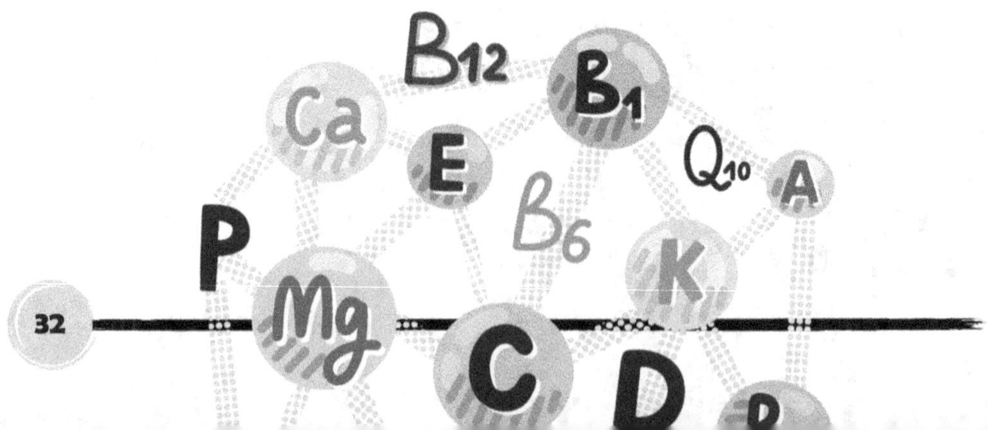

By adapting our intake of macronutrients, we can create a caloric deficit, since these are what provide our body with energy.

This adaptation affects both the quantitative aspect (caloric deficit) and the qualitative aspect.

It's not a question of randomly reducing our nutritional intake. The ratio between the different macronutrient groups (proteins, carbohydrates, lipids) is crucial.

For the same quantity by weight, the different macronutrients will not have the same caloric intake, nor provide us with the same nutritional components. Our bodies will therefore not process them in the same way.

Micronutrient intake should not be overlooked either, as it will have a major impact on our body's ability to function properly.

Let's take a closer look at the role and impact of macronutrients on our bodies.

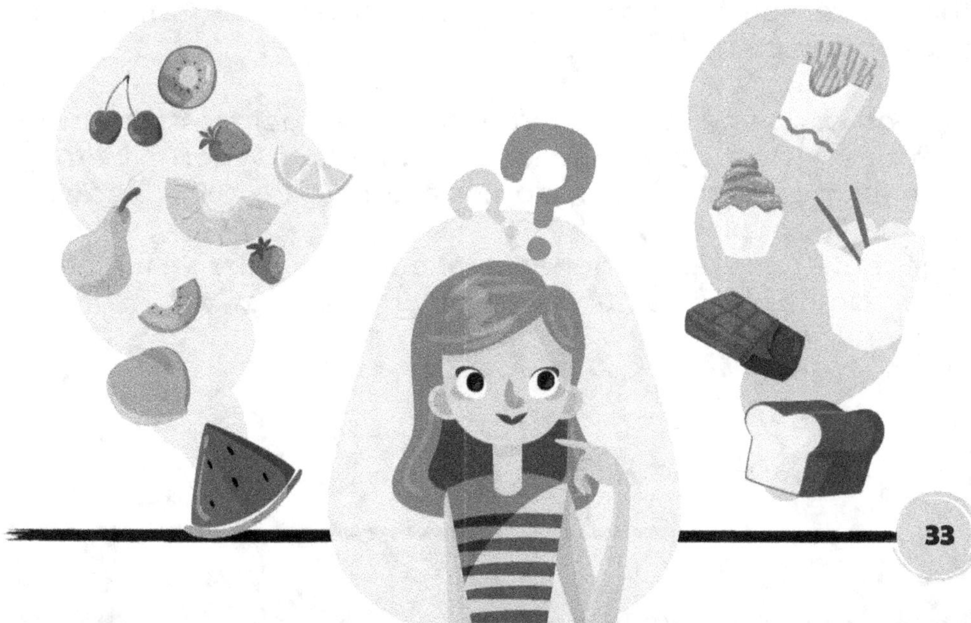

MACRONUTRIENTS

Proteins

Proteins are made up of amino acids, which are molecules composed mainly of carbon, hydrogen, nitrogen and oxygen.

Proteins are essential for building and maintaining our tissues. They are the main components of our muscles, skin and hair.

In fact, it's the second most important component of the human body, after water. It's also important to know that, unlike carbohydrates and lipids, our bodies can't store proteins.

In our diet, proteins can be of either animal or plant origin.

Animal proteins are found in meat, fish, eggs and dairy products.

Plant proteins are mainly found in cereals (wheat, oats...), legumes (kidney beans, lentils, chickpeas...), and oleaginous fruits (almonds, walnuts, seeds...).

There are some notable differences between animal and plant proteins.

Animal proteins contain more amino acids than plant proteins. That said, animal proteins also contain more fats (some of which can damage cardiovascular health if consumed in excess).
Vegetable proteins generally contain fiber, which is beneficial for digestion, and much less fat than animal proteins.

Carbohydrates

Carbohydrates are made up of carbon, hydrogen and oxygen.
They are our body's main source of energy.

During digestion, carbohydrates are first broken down into glucose, which is then absorbed into the bloodstream to supply energy to the various cells.

When this glucose is in excess, it is transformed into fatty acid, which is then stored as triglycerides (after further transformation) in adipose cells (i.e. fat).

There are two types of carbohydrate: simple and complex.

Simple carbohydrates (e.g. fructose, glucose, sucrose and lactose) are rapidly digested and cause a rapid rise in blood glucose levels. This level is called the Glycemic Index.

They are found, for example, in sugar, fruit, honey, candy, sweet drinks, cakes... In short, all sweet foods.

Complex carbohydrates (such as starch) are digested more slowly. They are found in starchy foods such as cereals, rice, potatoes and pasta. These carbohydrates generally don't taste sweet.

Simple carbohydrates have a higher glycemic index than complex carbohydrates.
In simple terms, a high glycemic index causes rapid digestion, and therefore an increase in blood glucose levels. This triggers a spike in insulin (the hormone that regulates glucose levels), which in turn converts excess glucose into fat.

Lipids

Lipids are also composed of carbon, hydrogen and oxygen.

The main function of lipids is energy storage, but they also play a vital role in the proper functioning of our bodies.
For example, they are important building blocks for cells, enable the assimilation of certain vitamins, and contribute to the proper functioning of hormones.

In terms of nutrition, there are two types of lipids: saturated fatty acids and unsaturated fatty acids.

Saturated fatty acids are generally of animal origin. They are found in fatty meats (such as red meats), deli meats and certain dairy products (butter, cheese, etc.). However, some vegetable fats, such as palm oil and coconut oil, contain very high levels of saturated fatty acids.

These fatty acids are not bad for our bodies, provided they are consumed sensibly. Excessive consumption, on the other hand, is detrimental to cardiovascular health (due in particular to the notorious "bad cholesterol") and does absolutely nothing to regulate body fat.

Unsaturated fatty acids are often of plant origin. They are found, for example, in oleaginous fruits (from which oil can be extracted) such as avocados and olives, nuts (walnuts, almonds...), and seeds (sunflower, sesame, flax...). Of course, the oils derived from these oilseeds also contain unsaturated fatty acids.

Some legumes, such as peanuts and soy, also contain high levels of unsaturated fatty acids.

Finally, these fatty acids are also found in certain fish (known as oily fish), such as salmon, mackerel, sardines, herring, sea bass, sea bream...

Unsaturated fatty acids are good for your health, and pose few risks. On the contrary, they are highly beneficial to the cardiovascular system. In fact, this family includes Omega 3, 6 and 9, which are fatty acids that are highly beneficial to our bodies.

Here's a relatively simple tip for identifying fatty acids: Saturated fatty acids are generally solid at room temperature, like butter or animal fat. Unsaturated fatty acids, on the other hand, are generally liquid at room temperature, like vegetable oil, and don't set in the fridge.

There are exceptions. Coconut oil, for example, is classified as a saturated fatty acid, even though it is liquid at room temperature.

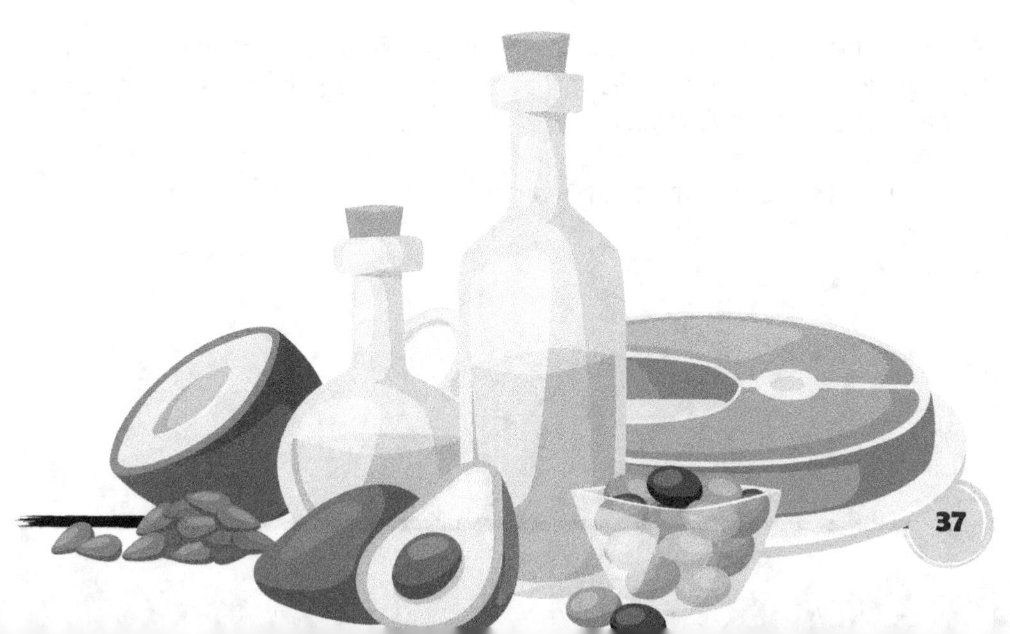

MICRONUTRIENTS

Vitamins

Vitamins are nutrients with no calorific value. They are nevertheless very important for the proper functioning of our metabolism.

Among other things, they are involved in blood circulation, immune system function, the nervous system and cell growth.

They fall into two broad categories:
Fat-soluble vitamins and water-soluble vitamins.

Fat-soluble vitamins include vitamins A, D, E and K.

They are found in fat-rich foods such as oily fish, oils, dairy products, eggs, meat and offal, as well as in certain fruits and vegetables, such as carrots, green leafy vegetables and apricots.

Vitamin D can also be synthesized by the body through exposure to sunlight.

Water-soluble vitamins are vitamins C and B.

They are found in water-rich foods, whether fruit (oranges, strawberries, etc.) or vegetables (broccoli, cereals, legumes, etc.).

Meat is also a source of vitamin B.

Minerals and trace elements

Minerals and trace elements are actually atoms of different natures, necessary for proper organic functioning. The only difference between minerals and trace elements is the quantity present in the body. Minerals are present in greater quantities than trace elements.

The most important minerals and trace elements are calcium, magnesium, phosphorus, potassium, copper, iron, fluorine, iodine, manganese, zinc and selenium.

Minerals and trace elements can be found just about everywhere: in water, plant products (vegetables, cereals, fruit) and animal products (meat, fish, seafood)... And even in dark chocolate (magnesium).

Probiotics

Probiotics are living micro-organisms, such as certain beneficial bacteria.

Probiotics play an important role in digestion and the immune system. Recent studies have also demonstrated the link between digestive health (which is greatly influenced by probiotics) and mental health.

Probiotics are found in fermented dairy products (yoghurts, cheeses), certain fermented foods (such as sauerkraut), and certain fermented beverages (such as kombucha).

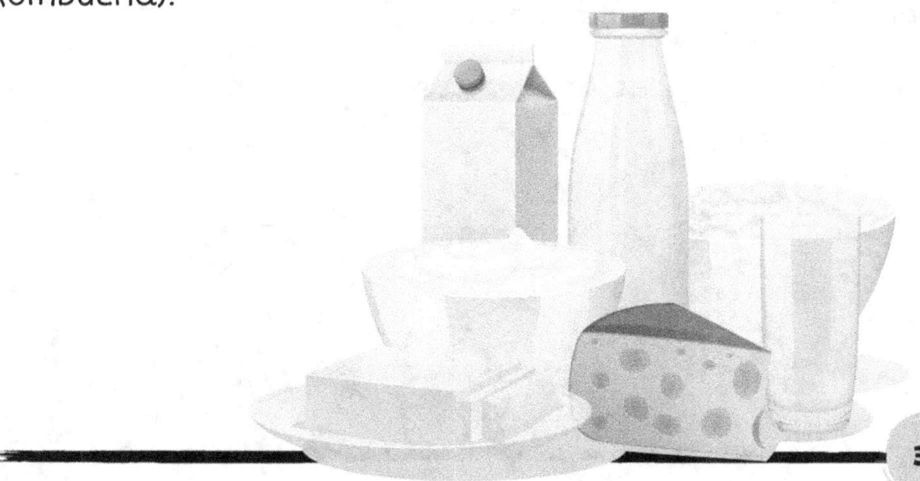

OTHER ELEMENTS

In addition to macronutrients and micronutrients, there are other elements that form part of our diet.

Dietary fiber

Dietary fibers are elements of plant origin that resist digestion in the stomach and small intestine.

They play an important role in the proper functioning of the colon (large intestine). They improve intestinal transit by acting on stool consistency, intestinal contraction and bacterial activity (through fermentation). They also have a positive effect on satiety.

Fiber, on its own, has a derisory caloric intake.

It is found in fruit, vegetables, legumes and wholegrain cereals.

Water

Water is essential to our bodies, and plays a part in a number of important processes, such as hydration, blood circulation, body temperature regulation, waste elimination and digestion.

Water is also a source of certain minerals, such as calcium, sodium and magnesium.

Water alone provides no calories.

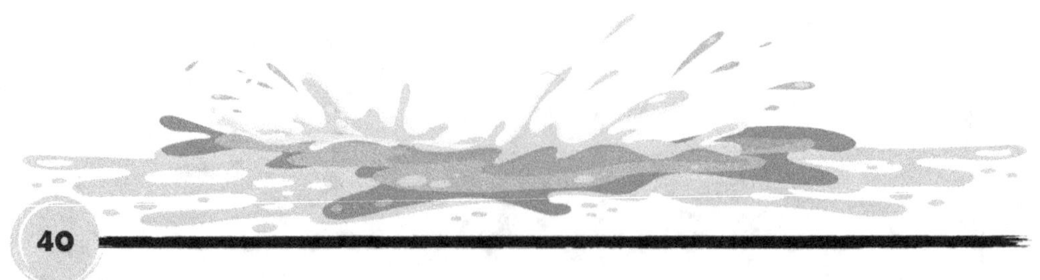

Antioxidants

Simply put, antioxidants are molecules that protect our cells from premature aging.

Certain vitamins (A, C, E) play an antioxidant role, as do certain minerals (zinc, selenium). The antioxidant family also includes other complex molecules, such as polyphenols.

Their caloric intake is negligible.

They are found in berries, citrus fruit, vegetables, nuts, oily fish, certain spices (turmeric, saffron), green tea, coffee and dark chocolate.

Sweeteners

Sweeteners are sugar substitutes. They are substances or food additives that have a sweet taste.

Honey and maple syrup can be considered natural sweeteners. Most sweeteners, however, are synthetic (non-natural) elements that provide a sweet taste while limiting caloric intake.

The trouble is, their impact on our health is not yet well known. Some studies even show that certain synthetic sweeteners present cardiovascular and neurological risks.

Most low-calorie products (soft drinks, foods from the food industry) contain artificial sweeteners.

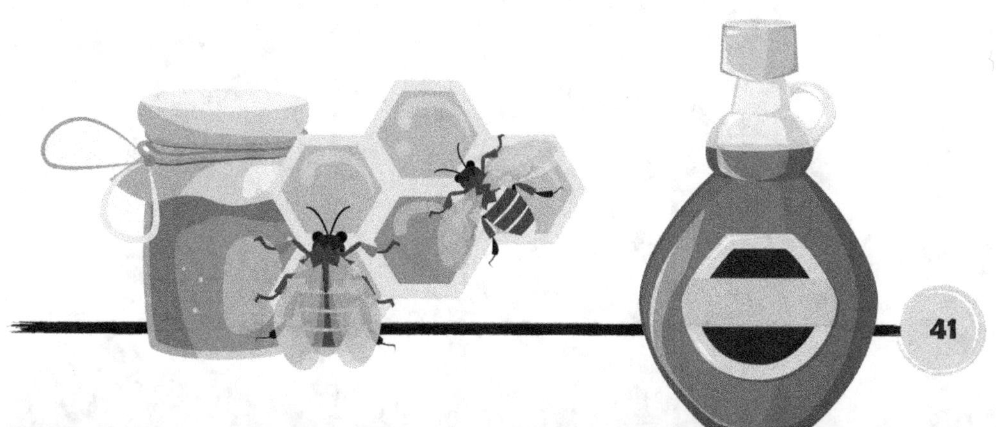

Food additives

Food additives are substances added to food to improve taste, color, texture or preservation.

They are found, in greater or lesser quantities, in processed food products (i.e. those produced by the food industry). These include ready-made meals, sweets, soft drinks, industrial cakes, etc. It is estimated that around 80% of industrial foods contain additives.

They have little or no calorie content.

Some additives are of natural origin, such as citric acid or chlorophyll. But most additives are synthetically produced, and again, some have little-known effects on our bodies.

Studies have shown that some additives can provoke allergic reactions, as well as risks of cancer and endocrine disruption (i.e. dysfunction of the hormonal system).

Caffeine

Caffeine is a natural substance found in coffee, tea, cola and dark chocolate. It is also found in energy drinks.

Caffeine has a stimulating effect on the nervous system. It tends to improve concentration and alertness. It provides virtually no energy.

However, excessive consumption can lead to sleep disorders, digestive problems and anxiety.

Alcohol

Alcohol is also known as ethanol. It is a molecule composed of carbon, hydrogen and oxygen.

Alcohol has a psychoactive effect, i.e. it acts on the central nervous system, altering our mood, perception, consciousness and motor skills.

Other psychoactive substances include tobacco, cocaine, doping products and certain medications (psychotropic drugs).

Some alcohols, such as red wine, have positive effects, as they contain antioxidants.

However, the harmful effects are not negligible. Excessive and regular consumption of alcohol poses risks to the liver, digestive system, heart and pancreas, not to mention the risk of dependency.

Last but not least, alcohol is very high in calories. Strong alcohols (whisky, rum...) have a very high energy intake, 4 to 5 times higher than a milder alcohol such as beer. But all this has to be seen in relation to the quantities consumed, and any other products mixed in (as with cocktails).

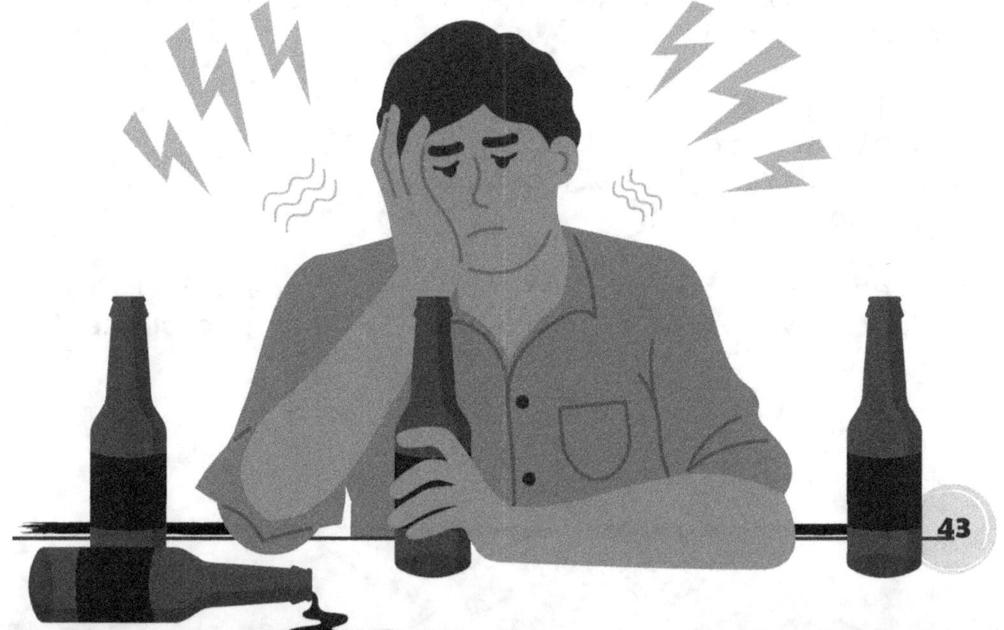

HOW TO CALCULATE CALORIES

We've just seen that not all nutrients have the same impact on our bodies.

Energy intake only comes from macronutrients, as well as alcohol (which is not a nutrient).

It's important, especially when you want to lose body fat, to estimate your total daily energy intake.

This total, as we have seen, should be related to our TDEE (total energy expenditure).

In simple terms, if the total calories in our diet exceed our TDEE, then we're going to store body fat. If this total is equal to our TDEE, then our body fat will be stable. And if this total is less than our TDEE, we create a caloric deficit, forcing our body to draw energy from our reserves (fat).

So let's start by learning how to calculate the calories in our diet.

There are several ways of doing this.

The first is to take the calorie bases of each macronutrient.

These bases are :
Protein: 4 Kcal per gram.
Carbohydrates: 4 Kcal per gram.
Fat: 9 Kcal per gram.

This represents around 113 Kcal per ounce for proteins and carbohydrates, and around 255 Kcal per ounce for fats.

This method is effective, but sometimes complicated to implement.

It's important to understand that a food is rarely 100% composed of a single macronutrient.

Take, for example, a 100-gram (3.5 Oz) portion of roast chicken breast. There's no question of doing the following calculation: 100 grams (3.5 Oz) X 4 Kcal = 400 Kcal. That would be a false estimate.

The average chicken breast contains 27 grams of protein and 1.5 grams of fat. The amount of carbohydrates is zero.

You'd have to do the following calculation: (27 grams (protein) X 4 Kcal) + (1.5 grams (fat) X 9 Kcal) = 121.5 Kcal.

This method is therefore very precise, but requires a lot of calculations for a single product. It also requires knowledge of the macronutrient composition of each food.

A slightly simpler method is to refer to nutrition tables, which give the calorie content (per 100 grams or 3.5 Oz) of most foods.

Of course, these are estimates, and the number of calories may vary according to the exact composition of the food, or its cooking method.

Nutrition tables are appended to this book.

They list most common foods, classified by type, and give an estimate of calorie intake and macronutrient proportions.

For dishes composed of several foods and made at home by ourselves, such as lasagne or a cake, we'll need to add up the caloric intake of each element, according to its quantity.

For example, if we make a cake with one egg, 150 grams (5.3 Oz) of flour, 100 grams (3.5 Oz) of chocolate, and 100 grams (3.5 Oz) of butter and 50 grams (1.75 Oz) of sugar, we'll need to calculate the calorie intake of one egg, then 150 grams of flour, then 100 grams of chocolate, and so on.

Then add up all the values, and divide by the number of servings.

Of course, once again, this is only an estimate, as cooking methods can slightly alter calorie intake.

For industrial products and foods, we recommend that you refer to the labels on the packaging, which indicate the product's nutritional values.

In any case, whatever method you use, you're going to have to weigh your food, or estimate its weight fairly precisely.

And each food must be taken into account. For example, a dose of ketchup or a lump of sugar in coffee must be accounted for.

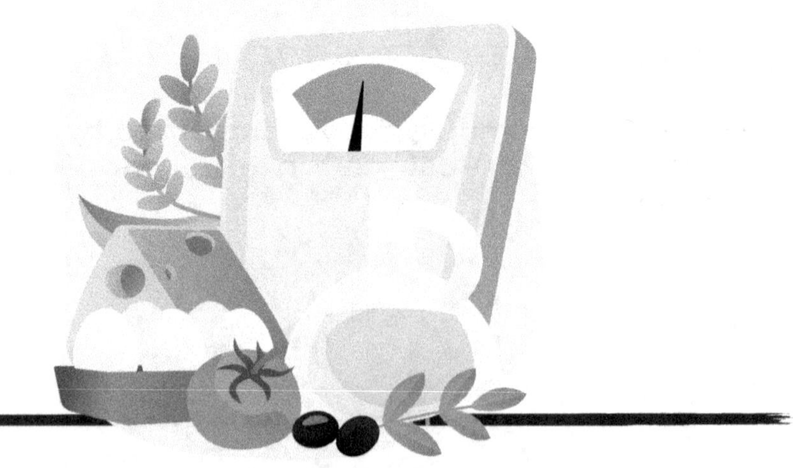

HOW TO WEIGH FOOD

To calculate our energy intake, we need to calculate the quantity of food consumed. This quantity is generally calculated by weight (in grams), and sometimes by volume for beverages.

The most efficient way to do this is to weigh each food item on a scale, and record the corresponding number of Kcal.

Then add these numbers together to obtain the total calories consumed in a meal. And so on for each meal. At the end of the day, we obtain our total energy intake.

Let's take an example with a meal consisting of 100 grams (3.5 Oz) of salmon (200 Kcal), 100 grams (3.5 Oz) of white rice (150 Kcal) and 100 grams (3.5 Oz) of broccoli (35 Kcal).
This gives us a total of 385 Kcal.

This method is the most efficient, and provides a relatively accurate estimate of our calorie intake. But it is also somewhat restrictive.

You have to weigh each food item, and that's not always possible. For example, how can we weigh our food when we're not at home?

And let's face it, our days can get pretty full, and we can forget to weigh our food, or simply skip it for lack of time and energy.

Fortunately, there's a trick to estimating the weight of food. And for this, we're going to use our hand.

In theory, a palm-sized portion of protein-rich food (meat, fish, etc.) should be around 100-150 grams (3.5/5.3 Oz). A portion of carbohydrate-rich foods (rice, pasta) the size of our closed fist should also be around 100/150 grams. And finally, a thumb-sized portion of lipid-rich products (butter, oil) represents around 15/20 grams (0.5/0.7 Oz).

These measurements are theoretical, as they depend on the size of our hand, but also on the density of the food.

For a more precise estimate, simply cut a piece of meat the size of your palm (note that the thickness must be almost identical), and weigh it. This gives us a more precise estimate of the weight equivalent to our palm. We then do the same, weighing a quantity of pasta or rice the size of our fist, and a quantity of butter or oil equivalent to our thumb.

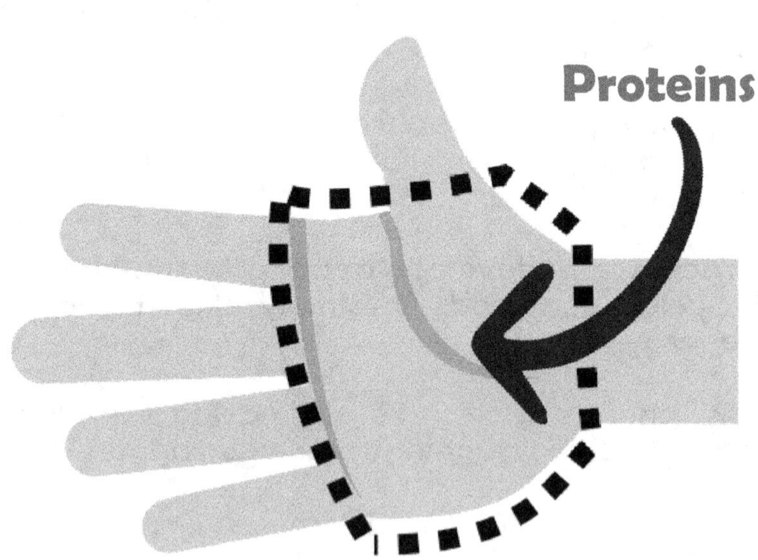

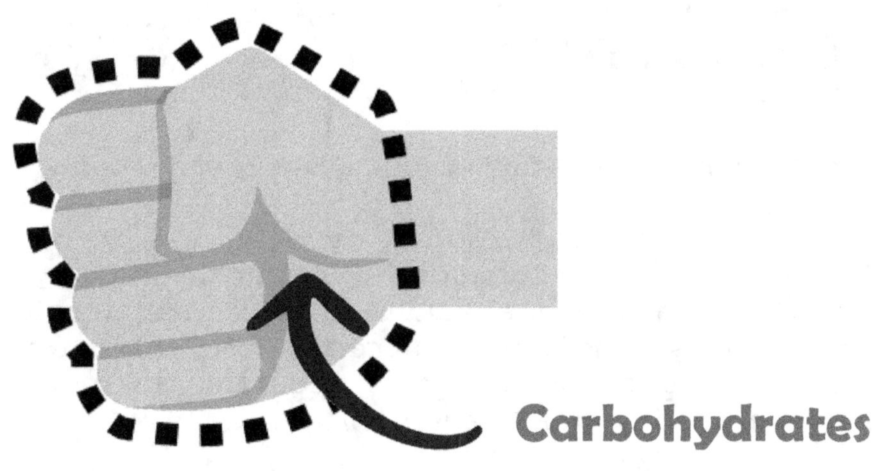

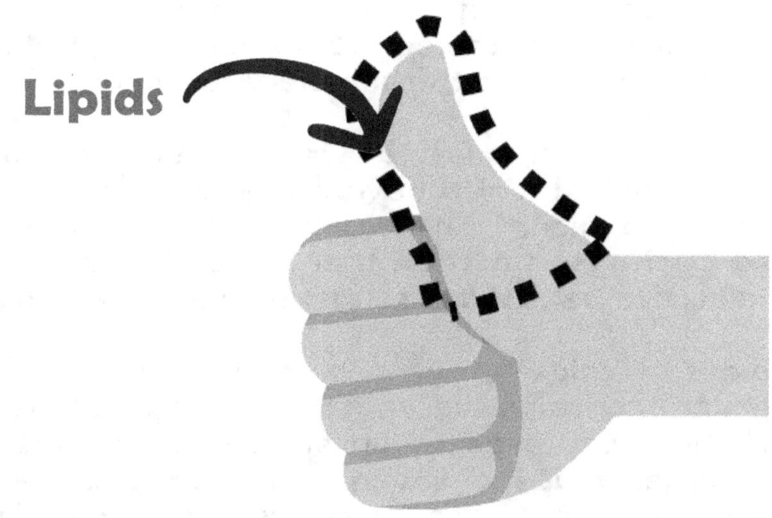

Now we can estimate the weight of our food without taking out the scales!

Let's try to calculate our calorie intake over a few days, without changing our eating habits. Compare them with our TDEE.

By how many Kcal are we exceeding our TDEE?

FOOD QUALITY

Now we know how to estimate our daily energy intake.

From a purely quantitative point of view, and in theory, all we need to do is calculate our caloric intake and reduce the quantities we swallow to create a caloric deficit. But unless the aim is to create deficiencies and a constant feeling of hunger, this reduction in quantity alone doesn't really make sense.

Let's take a simple example. A fast-food hamburger (250 grams or 8.8 Oz) has an energy value of around 450 Kcal. A meal consisting of chicken (100g or 3.5 Oz), rice (100g) and cooked vegetables (100g) with vegetable oil and yoghurt has almost the same energy value.

The hamburger is a major source of simple carbohydrates, which have a high glycemic index. It also contains a significant amount of saturated fats and food additives. On the other hand, it contains virtually no dietary fiber, and is relatively low in micronutrients.

A plate of chicken, rice and vegetables, accompanied by yoghurt, contains very little saturated fat, and the carbohydrates present (in smaller quantities than in a hamburger) have a lower glycemic index. We also find more fiber and micronutrients, and only yogurt may contain a few additives.

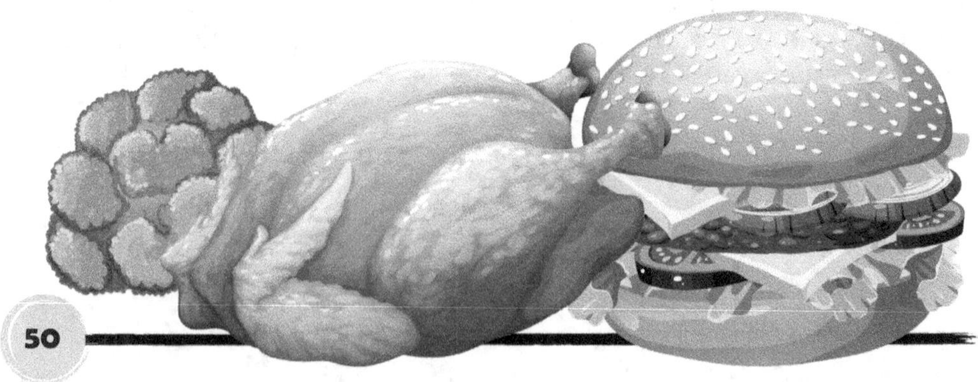

In conclusion, a hamburger and a plate of chicken/rice/vegetables have the same energy value (450 Kcal) but not at all the same nutritional value.

Which of these meals do you think is most likely to promote fat storage? The hamburger or the chicken plate?

Let's take another example. A 12 Oz (36 cl) bottle of beer is worth around 150 Kcal. That's the same energy value as a 160g banana. Do you think that beer has the same nutritional value as a banana?

Caloric values are important, but they're only an indicator. In other words, yes, they need to be calculated or estimated, but they're not the only parameter to take into account.

This brings us to the qualitative aspect of our diet.

Sometimes, if you're just a little overweight, simply readjusting your diet to make it healthier is enough to trigger fat loss.

For example, replacing foods that are far too rich in simple carbohydrates with healthier ones can result in a calorie deficit for the same amount of food. 100 grams (3.5 Oz) of banana are worth an average of 90 Kcal, but 100 grams (3.5 Oz) of cookies are generally worth over 500 Kcal. In conclusion, replacing cookies with a banana can create a deficit of over 400 Kcal.

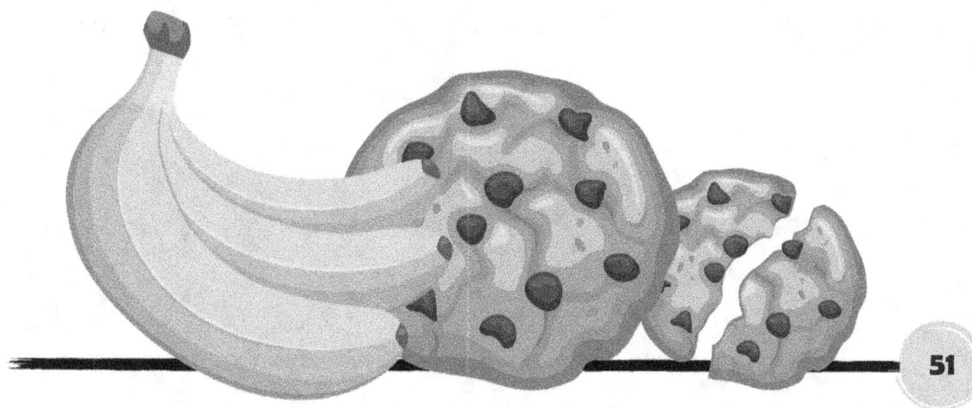

CALORIC DEFICIT

Now that we know how to calculate our energy intake and are aware of the importance of food quality, let's take a look at how to create a caloric deficit.

As we have seen, this deficit will force our body to draw on our fat reserves. However, it's not a question of doing just anything, anyhow.

If we create a large caloric deficit too quickly, chances are our body won't react very well. We'll feel tired, hungry and hard to control, and we'll probably be in a bad mood. This is what most restrictive diets cause.

Conversely, if the caloric deficit is insufficient, we won't lose any fat.

So let's proceed in stages.

The first thing to do is to create a balance between our energy needs and our energy expenditure. In other words, our caloric intake must be equal to our TDEE. To achieve this, we need to adopt a healthy, balanced diet, and calculate our daily intake. We'll also balance our macronutrient portions (see next page).

This first step will vary in duration, depending on our starting situation. The objective is as follows: In the first week, we're going to lower our calorie intake by 200 Kcal per day. The second week, we'll lower our intake by another 200 Kcal, and so on until our energy intake equals our TDEE.

In the second stage, we create a caloric deficit. Here again, the duration will vary according to our starting situation and goal.

For the first two or three weeks, we'll create a caloric deficit of 150 to 300 Kcal per day. Of course, we'll always pay close attention to the quality of our food.

At the end of this period, it's time to take stock. If we have started to achieve satisfactory results, we can maintain this deficit as it is.
If the results are not satisfactory (i.e. if we've lost very little body fat), we can again increase our deficit by 100 to 200 Kcal.

However, there are two points to bear in mind: Firstly, losing weight takes time. We can't expect to lose all our belly fat in 2 weeks. It's a process that takes time and patience. Secondly, before creating a caloric deficit again, I invite you to read the section devoted to physical activity (which is also an excellent way of creating or increasing the caloric deficit).

To help us keep track of our daily intake, a blank table is included in the appendix of this book.

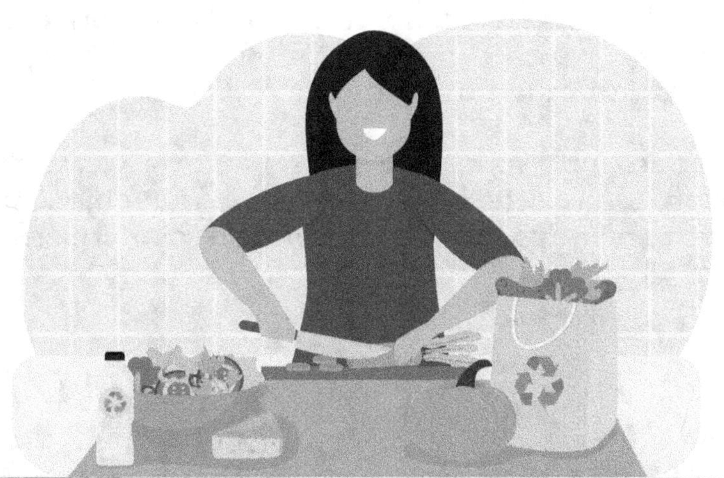

MACRONUTRIENT RATIO

Precisely calculating the right ratio between macronutrients is no simple matter. A multitude of parameters need to be taken into account, such as gender and age, but also the objective (e.g. weight loss), and physical activity. Finally, our morphology and metabolism play an important role.

You should also be aware that there are no magic formulas, and that we can find very different ratios (on the Internet, for example) for the same objective.

For a person with little physical activity and wishing to lose weight, we will use the following ratios:

Protein: 30 to 35%.
Carbohydrates: 45 to 50%.
Fat: 15 to 20%.

Protein is important for muscle maintenance, so we're going to encourage this.

Lipids are important for proper hormonal and cellular functioning. Be careful, however, as this macronutrient group is quite high in calories.

Carbohydrates are our body's main source of energy. We will therefore be focusing on this group to create a caloric deficit. We'll also be focusing on complex carbohydrates, and limiting simple carbohydrates (sugary foods) as much as possible.

Generally speaking, to refine these ratios according to our situation, we will base ourselves on our objective (the amount of fat mass to be lost) and our intensity of physical activity.

For sports enthusiasts, for example (even newcomers), it is possible to increase the protein ratio (10% maximum), and lower the carbohydrate ratio.

Now we need to convert these ratios into grams. To do this, we'll take into account our calorie target, i.e. the total number of calories we need to consume per day. This number will be equivalent to our TDEE if we're in the balance phase, and less than our TDEE if we're in the caloric deficit phase.

Here's the calculation, taking as an example an intake of 1800 Kcal and the following ratios:
Protein: 35
Carbohydrates: 45
Fat: 20%.

Protein: 1800 X 35 % = 630 Kcal
Carbohydrates: 1800 X 45 % = 810 Kcal
Fat: 1800 X 20% = 360 Kcal

In this example, we would need to consume 630 Kcal of protein, 810 Kcal of carbohydrates and 360 Kcal of fat.

It's important to understand that we must take macronutrients into account, and not the total weight of the food.
For example, a 100-gram (3.5 Oz) portion of steamed salmon contains 20 grams (0.7 Oz) of protein (or 80 Kcal), and 13 grams of fat (or 117 Kcal).

This macronutrient breakdown method is therefore relatively precise, but also rather complex.

Let's take a look at another, simpler method, just as effective for most of us.

It's all about dividing up the food on our plate.

So we're going to divide the food up as follows:
1/4 protein sources.
1/4 carbohydrate sources (complex).
1/2 vegetables.

This is the basis for the composition of our lunch and dinner.

Next, we'll add a variety of foods, divided between breakfast, snacks and desserts: 1-2 dairy products (at least one of which should be fermented, such as yoghurt or cheese), fruit and sources of unsaturated fats (almonds, walnuts). Finally, vegetable oil (olive, sunflower) should be used for cooking.

Of course, this breakdown can be adapted to suit sporting activities.

For example, we can slightly increase our protein portion, and lower our carbohydrate portion.

Let's also try not to lower the proportion of vegetables. We can even increase it if necessary. Vegetables contain fiber and micronutrients, and are low in energy. Eating a large quantity of vegetables will also promote satiety.

Please note, however, that this method does not dispense us from calculating our calorie intake in order to adapt the quantities we eat.

If we follow this dietary composition and watch our calorie intake, we're well on the way to losing body fat.

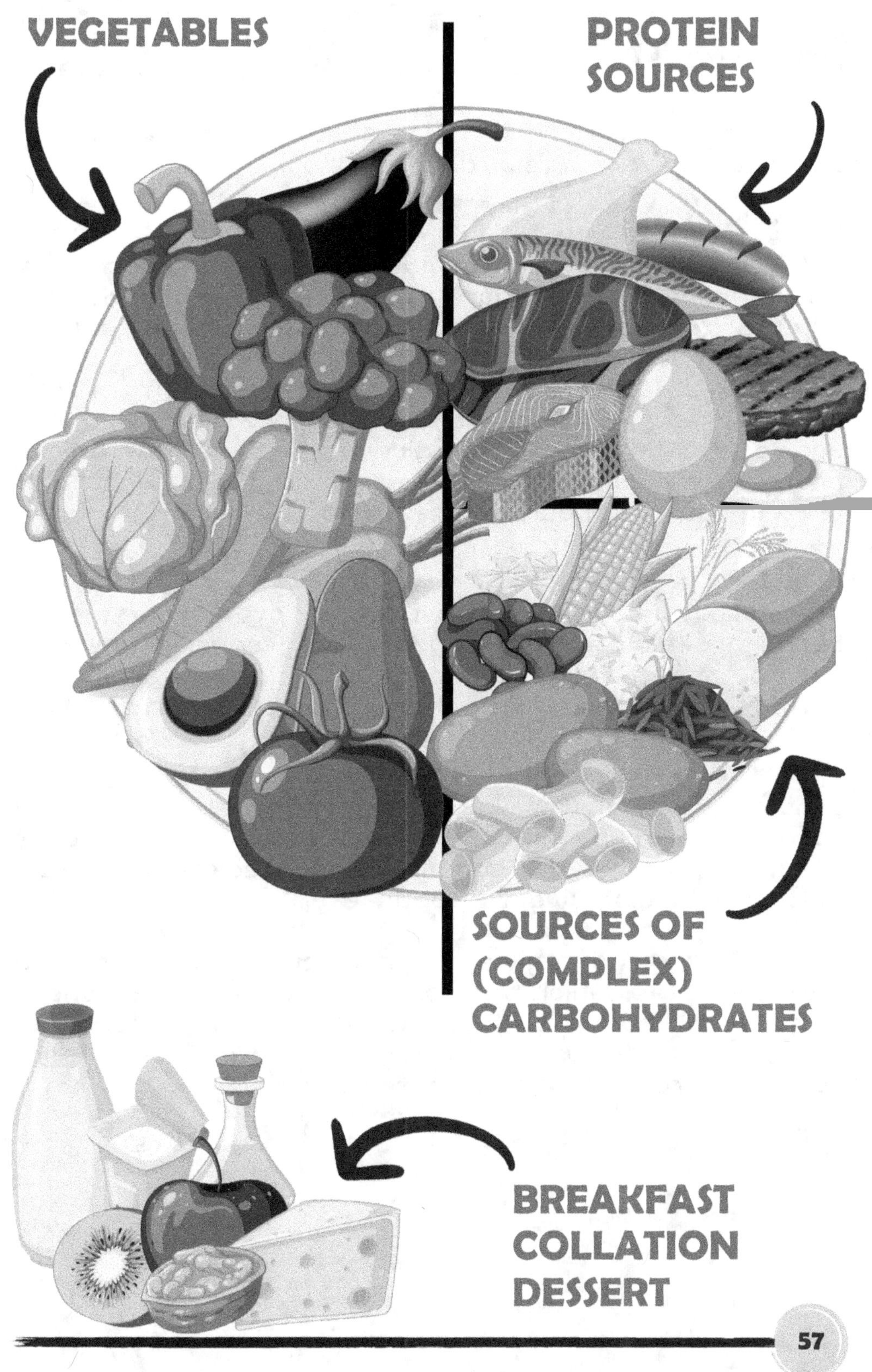

VEGETABLES
PROTEIN SOURCES
SOURCES OF (COMPLEX) CARBOHYDRATES
BREAKFAST COLLATION DESSERT

IMPORTANT RULES

Now that we know how to manage the composition of our diet, here are a few rules to follow.

Proteins

It's best to eat both animal and vegetable proteins. Animal proteins are more complete (amino acids) but often contain saturated fatty acids. Vegetable proteins contain fewer amino acids, but also very few saturated fatty acids. It is therefore advisable to diversify protein sources (meat, fish, cereals, legumes, etc.).
For vegetarians, eggs and dairy products contain animal proteins suitable for this diet. For vegans, vegetable protein sources should be as varied as possible.

Lipids

It's important to limit saturated fats (fatty meats, butter, cakes and other industrial products). Instead, opt for unsaturated fats of plant origin. Lean meats, with a fat content of less than 10%, are also preferable.

Carbohydrates

Simple carbohydrates, i.e. sugary foods, should be kept to a minimum. It is therefore necessary to reduce as much as possible the consumption of cakes (especially industrial cakes), sweets, sodas, etc....

We recommend giving preference to complex carbohydrates, which have a lower glycemic index, and in particular wholefoods such as wholegrain cereals, or products made with wholemeal flour. These foods contain more fiber and promote satiety.

Not forgetting...

Drastically limit alcohol, which provides a high energy intake and has recognized health risks. Limit sugary drinks too (fruit juices, syrups, soft drinks), and don't forget to include them in your macronutrient and calorie intake ratios.

Drink enough water, between 1 and 2 liters a day (33/67 Oz). Water hydrates our body and helps regulate our temperature. It is fundamental to the proper functioning of our organism. It also facilitates intestinal transit.

Plan your meals in advance to avoid impulsive food choices. This will also allow you to take the time to calculate the energy content of your diet.

Don't forget micronutrients, fiber and probiotics, by eating vegetables, fruit and dairy products.

Limit processed foods and dishes, which often contain food additives, as well as significant amounts of saturated fatty acids and sugar. Reading labels on this type of product will help you make better choices.

Diversify your menus. This helps avoid monotony.

Take time to eat, without outside distractions if possible (such as television, for example).

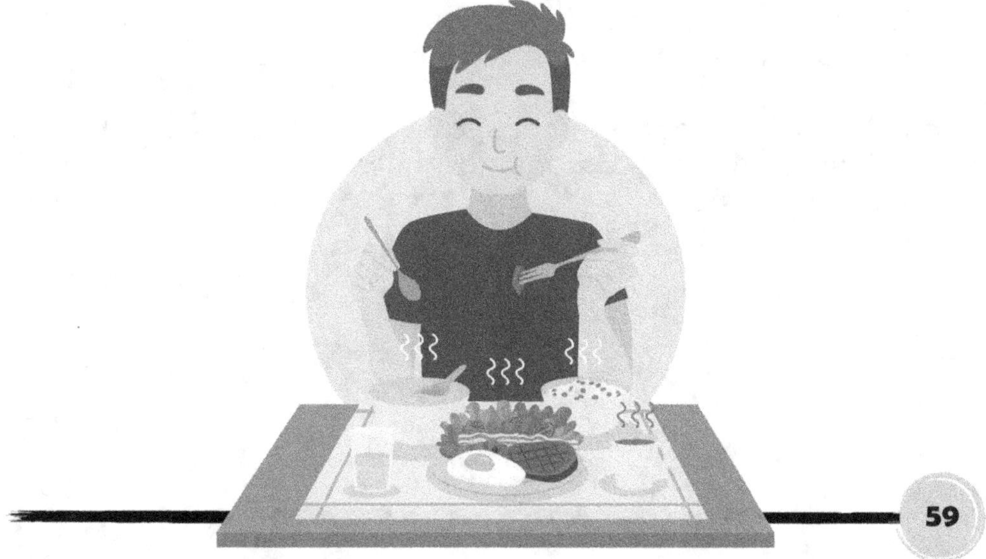

WHAT IF I'M HUNGRY?

Rebalancing your diet always requires effort. Sometimes our brains will encourage us to break the rules... but we mustn't give in.

Let's take an example to illustrate this. Sugar has an addictive effect on our brain. Indeed, when we eat a food with a high sugar content, our body secretes dopamine, which some scientists call "the pleasure molecule". Put simply, our brain interprets sugar as a reward. It therefore considers that it needs sugar frequently. But our bodies don't need sugar. This is just one example of how what we crave is not necessarily what we need.

But it's perfectly normal to feel the urge to eat outside of meals, to swallow a few pieces of chocolate, or to crave a large piece of cake as a snack. It's normal, but we have to fight these cravings, which are likely to ruin our efforts and have a detrimental effect on our fat loss.

And let's not forget to think about our goal, which will be a source of motivation to fight our urges.

So the first thing to do is to ask ourselves whether we're really hungry, or whether it's just a whim of our brain. To do this, we try to divert our brain's attention.

For example, we can concentrate on our work or on a TV show (especially not a cooking show!). And why not try a relaxation session?

We can also keep our hands busy (now's the time to do a jigsaw puzzle), or engage in physical activity (playing sports, mowing the lawn...).

If that's not enough, let's try fooling our brains by chewing gum. To avoid this having the opposite effect, it's best to take a mint (avoid fruity flavors) and sugar-free chewing gum.
Another tip is to brush your teeth. This sends a signal to the brain that it's no longer time to eat... And it's good for your teeth!

If, after 10 to 15 minutes, we still have that uncontrollable urge to eat, we can try drinking a large glass of water, tea or coffee (preferably with little or no sugar).

If the craving doesn't go away, hunger is probably real. But there's no question of getting out the packet of cookies! We can eat an apple (50 Kcal), a bowl of vegetable soup (around 100 Kcal), or a hard-boiled egg (75 Kcal). These foods have a significant satiating effect.

If we often feel hungry outside mealtimes, we'll probably need to readjust our food quantities, without increasing our energy intake.

To do this, we can increase our portion of vegetables, and increase the proportion of wholefoods in our carbohydrate intake.

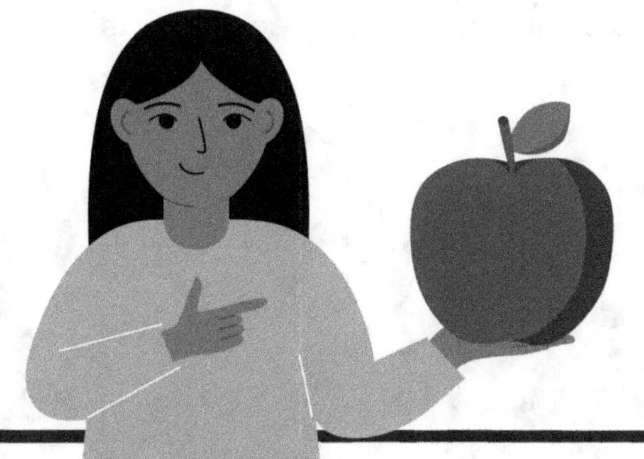

CHEAT MEALS

Cheat meals are meals where we allow ourselves a few pleasures and transgressions. They should be seen as a release valve, a moment when we can indulge in a tasty treat without worrying too much about energy intake.

But beware: a cheat meal must respect certain rules so as not to ruin our dietary efforts.

- It's a one-off meal or snack. Never have more than one cheat meal a week.

- It must be planned. You can't just decide to have a cheat meal because you've spotted a superb cake in a shop window.

- It has to be controlled. Even if we exceed our caloric intake and don't respect our macronutrient ratios, that's no reason to do just anything.

- It's not compulsory. If we've planned a cheat meal for tonight but don't really feel like it, that's okay! We'll make one in a few days.

Finally, here again, we're not all equal when it comes to these dietary deviations. So it's important to be aware of the repercussions.

The "cheat meal" rules also apply to the little pleasures we can indulge in on a more regular basis.

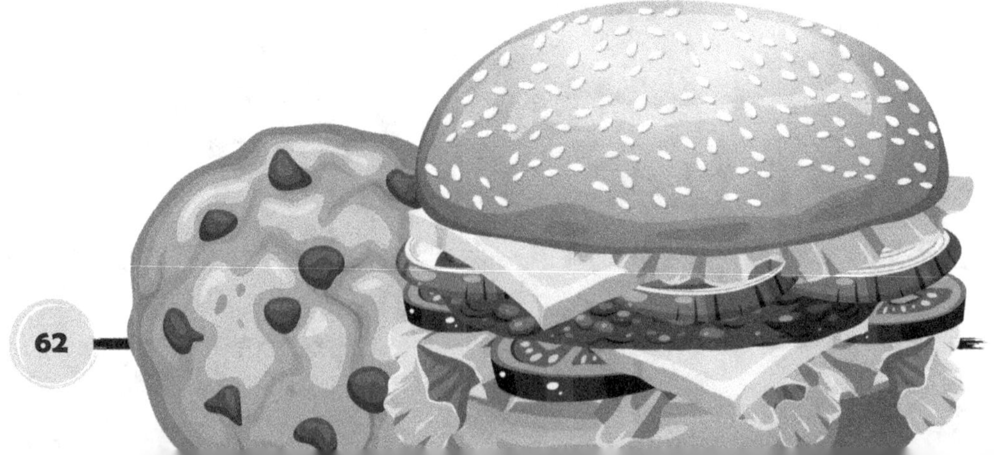

It's possible, for example, to eat a little chocolate every day, as long as you're reasonable about both quantity and quality. Preferably dark chocolate, with a reasonable sugar content.

Of course, you need to take into account your daily calorie intake, and avoid the accumulation of certain nutrients.

Chocolate, for example, contains sugar. We should therefore avoid any other overly sweet foods during the day.

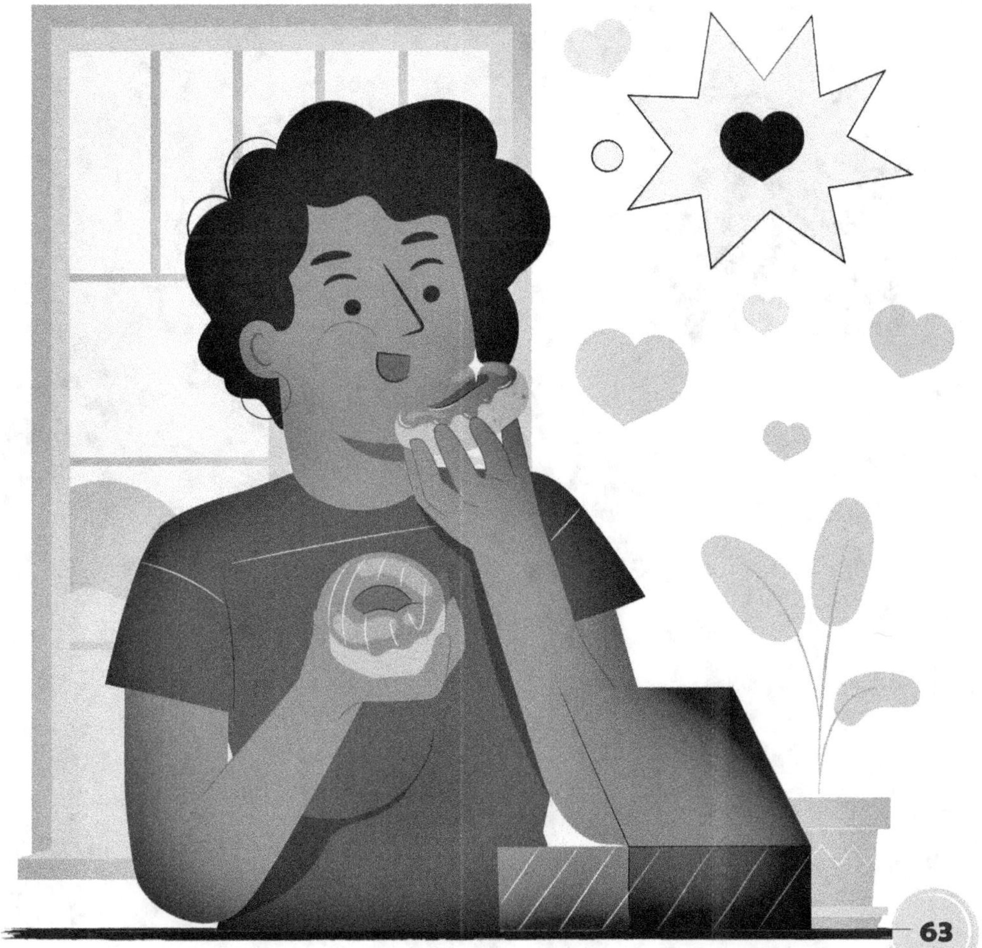

PHYSICAL ACTIVITY

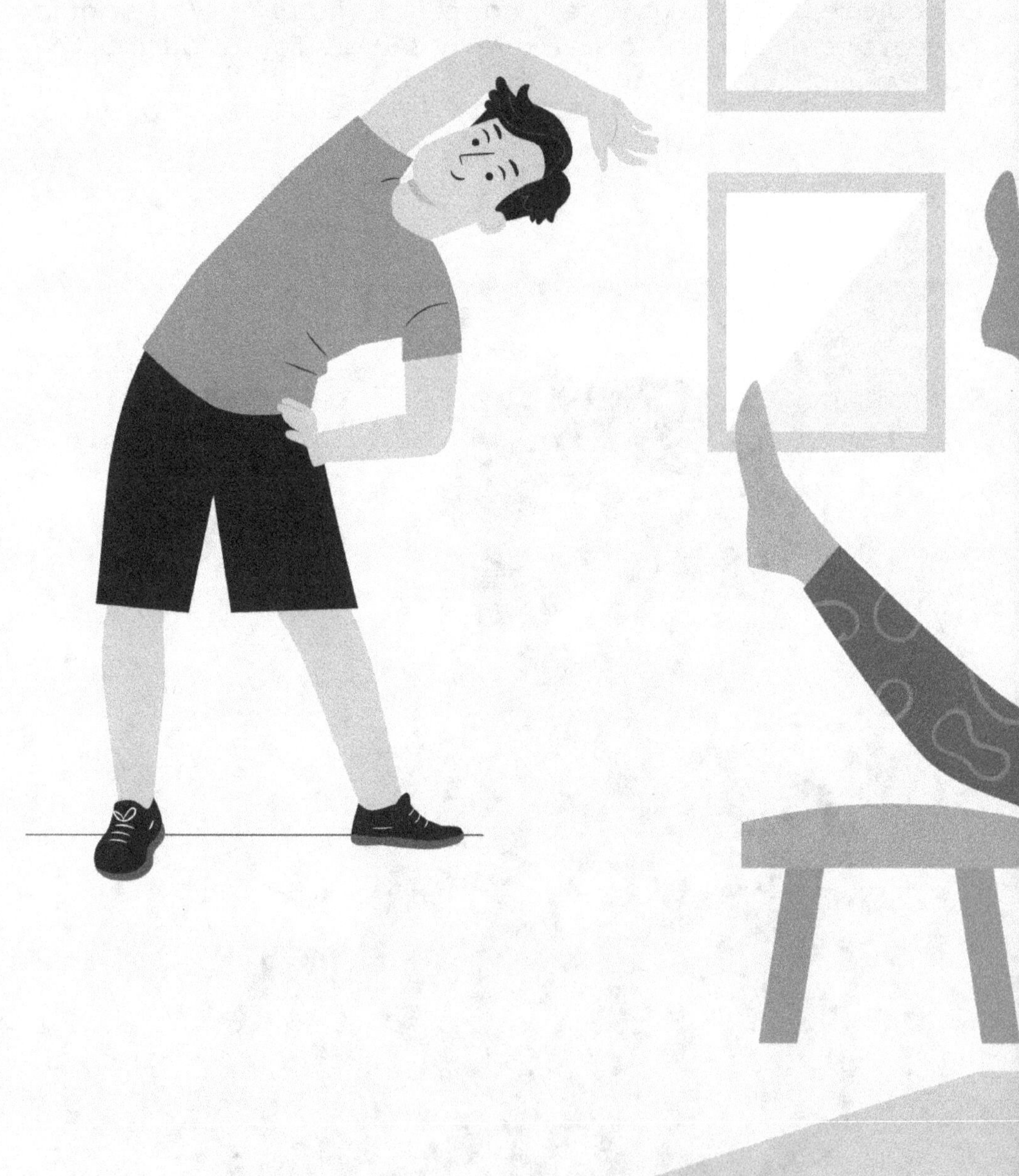

Like our diet, physical activity has a major impact on our health.

In this section, we'll look at a number of exercises we can use to tone our abdominal muscles and correct our posture.

We'll also look at physical activity from the angle of energy expenditure, and understand the impact of sleep and stress on fat accumulation.

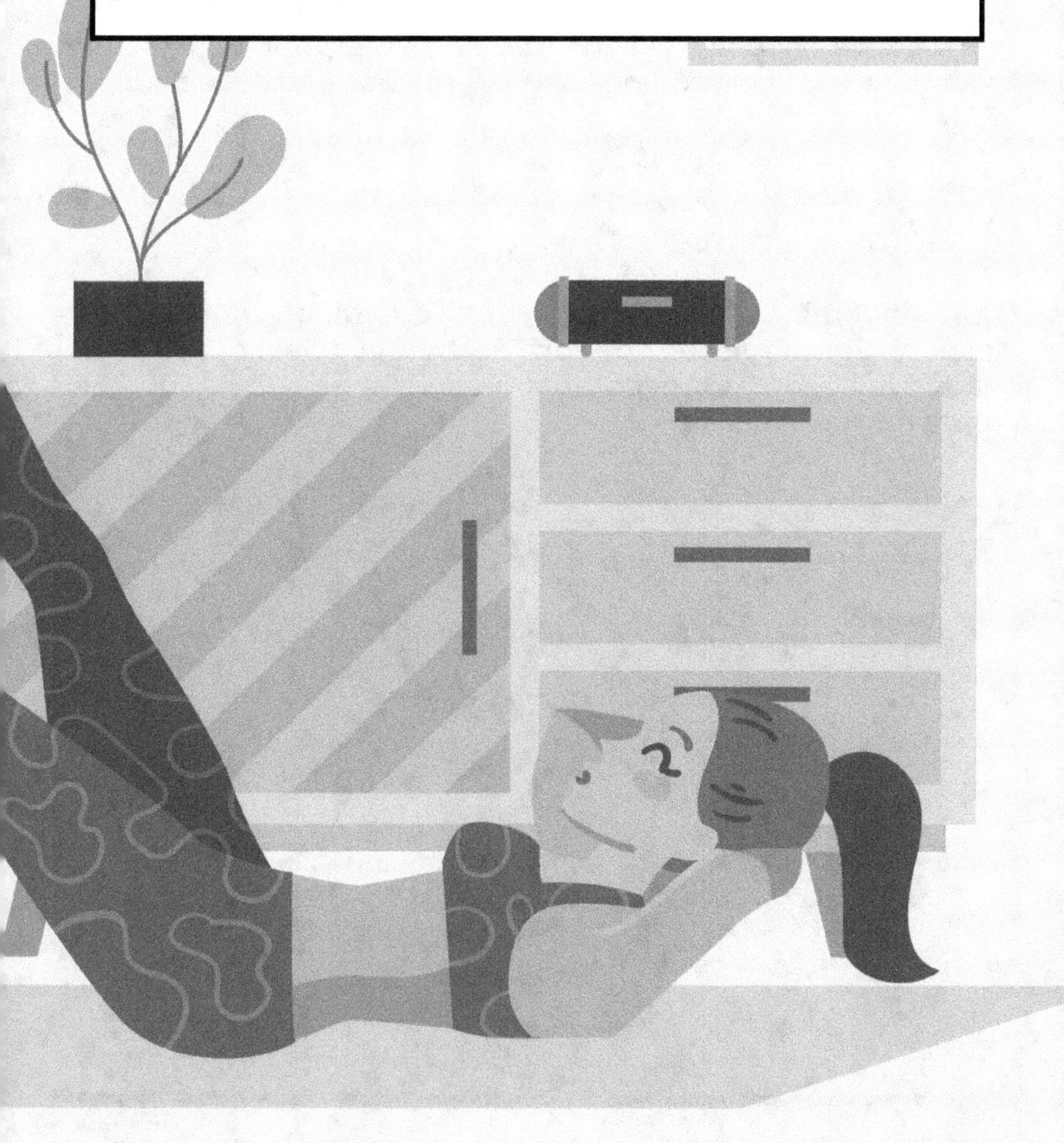

ABDOMINAL MUSCLES

The abdominal muscles are a very important muscle group.

Naturally, the first thing on our minds is aesthetics. Many of us dream of having visible abs (the famous six-pack).

But it's important to understand that the role of the abdominals goes far beyond aesthetics, as they contribute greatly to our posture... And poor posture can result in a protruding stomach, as we'll see in the following pages.

But first, let's take a look at the different abdominal muscles.

Our abdominal girdle (as the abdominal muscles are known) is made up of different muscles: the rectus abdominis, the external obliques, the internal obliques and the transverse.

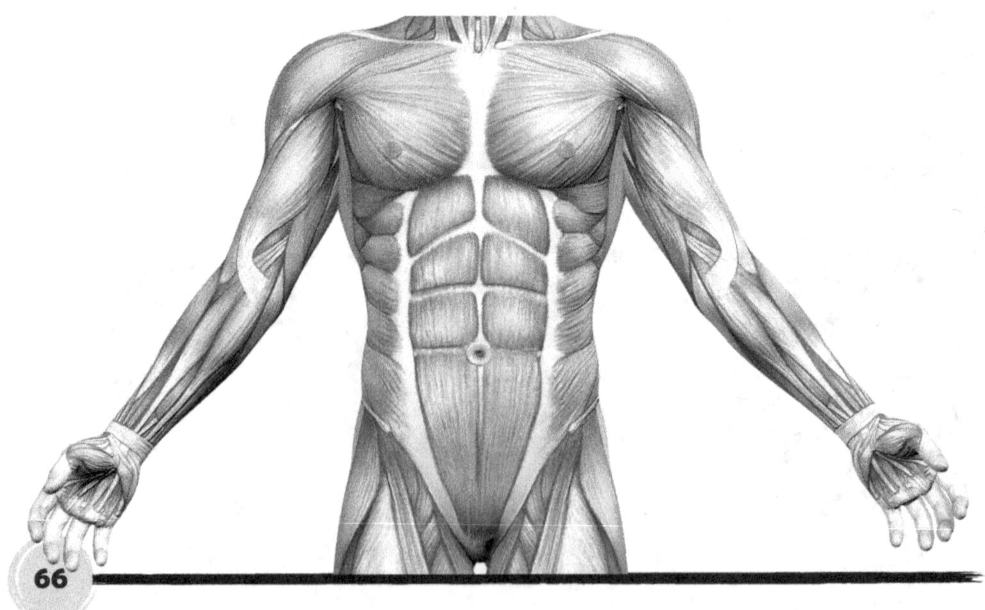

1. The rectus abdominis: This is the most obvious muscle, located at the front of the abdomen. Its main function is to tilt the trunk forward.
2. The external obliques: These are superficial muscles located on either side of the abdomen. They enable the trunk to tilt and rotate.
3. The internal obliques: These muscles are positioned laterally, below the external obliques, and also enable flexion and rotation of the trunk.
4. The transverse: This deep muscle acts like a corset to support the viscera in the abdominal cavity. It is the most important muscle for achieving a flat stomach.

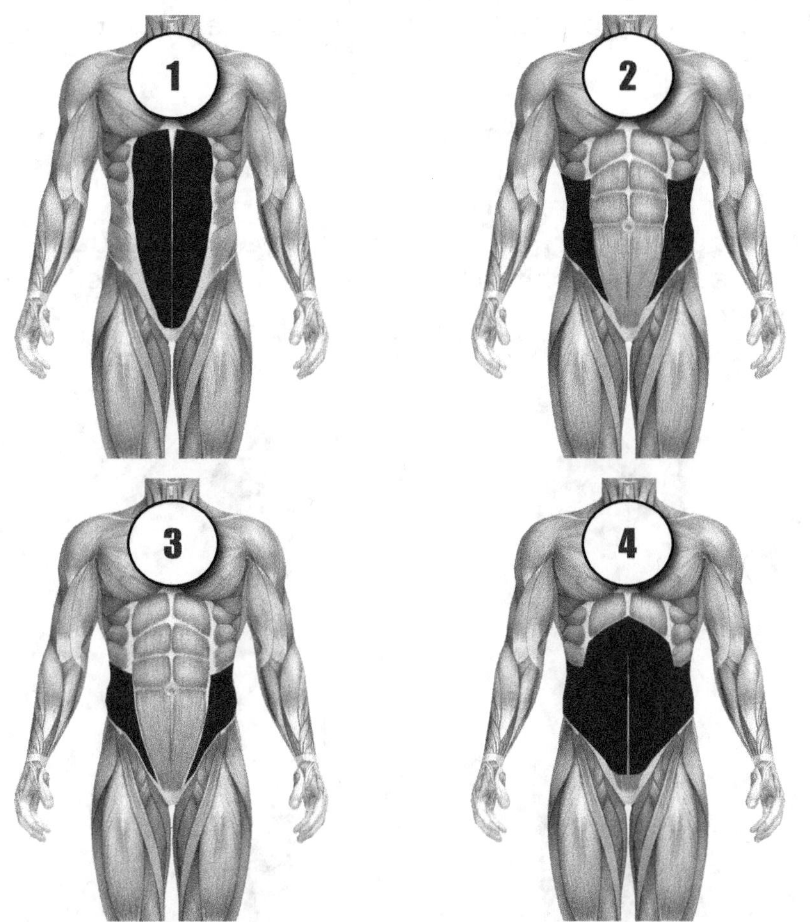

BACK POSTURE

As we've just seen, losing abdominal fat isn't enough to achieve a flat stomach. Our viscera exert pressure on our abdominal wall, and if our muscles aren't toned enough, they can't fight this pressure. In this case, our belly becomes slack and round.

Our general posture also has a major impact on the muscular relaxation of our belly. This is also true in the other direction: Muscular relaxation of the belly will have an impact on our general posture.

As far as we're concerned, we're going to look at the abnormal curvature of our spine (apart from any malformation or pathology requiring medical treatment, of course).

We can distinguish two main cases:
1. Accentuated arching of the lower back, known as lumbar hyperlordosis.
2. An accentuation of the curvature of the upper back (between the shoulder blades), known as thoracic hypercyphosis.

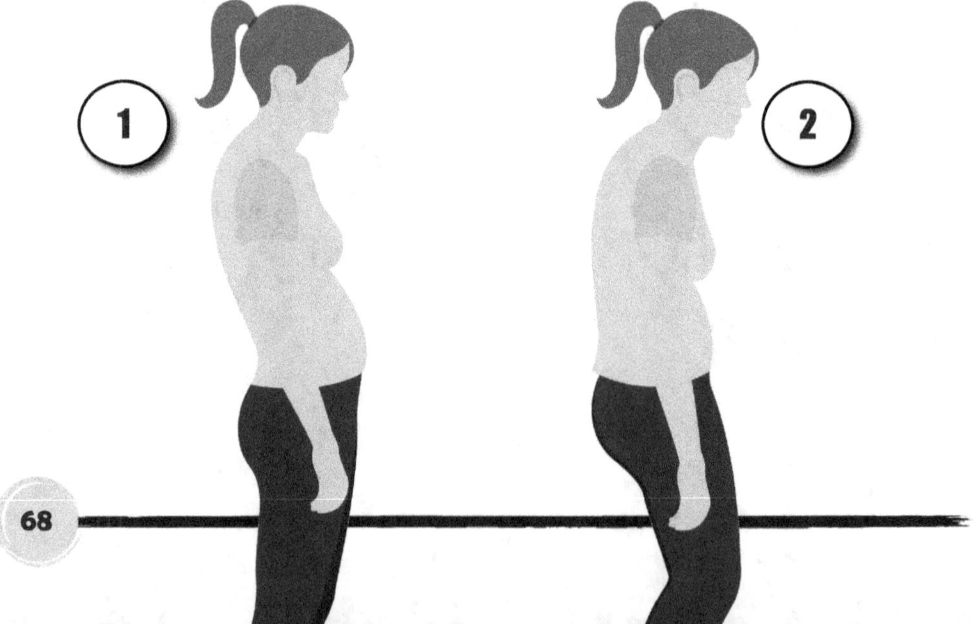

As we can see, these postural problems tend to make our belly stand out.

Of course, toning our abdominal muscles will have a beneficial effect on our posture, but that's not enough.

We also need to strengthen our back muscles, as they also play a very important role in maintaining good posture.

We're going to focus on the deep muscles that support our spine.

But first, let's start by adopting good posture habits.

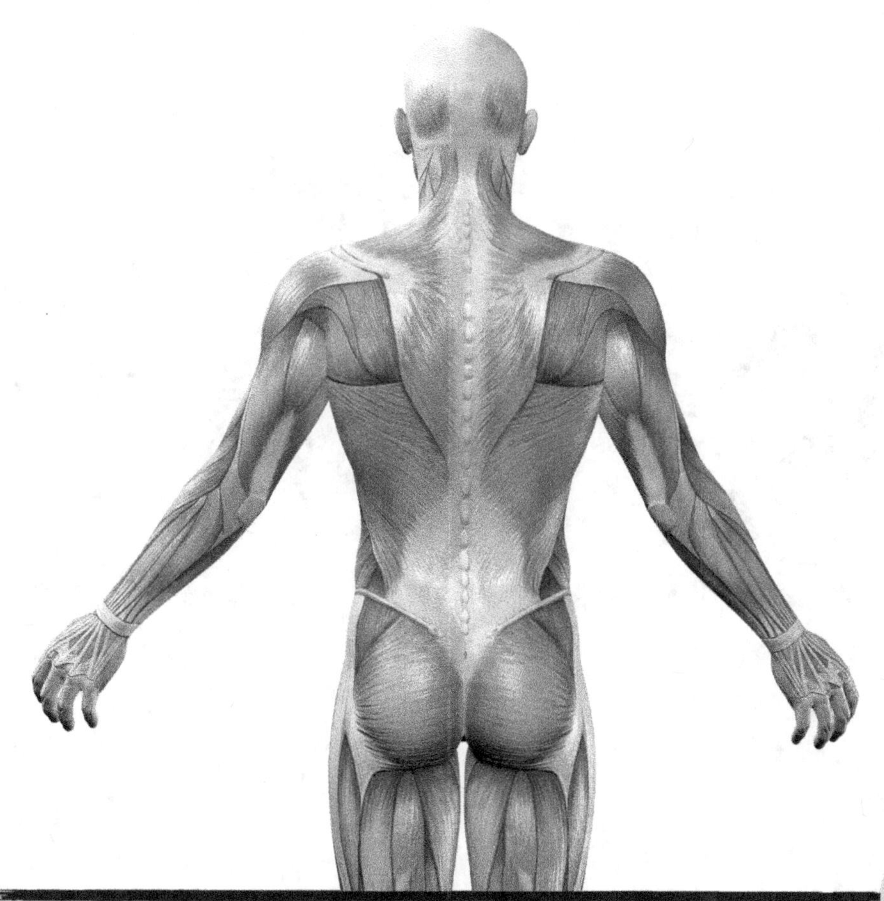

Very often, it's our bad daily habits that lead to bad posture.

All too often, for example, we sit hunched over in front of our computer. This is also the case when we stare at our phones for hours on end.

For women, high-heeled shoes tend to dig into the lower back.

So the first thing to do to improve our posture is to change our habits:
*   Stand and sit up straight. Keep shoulders back and head upright (to avoid stooping).
*   Wear shoes without heels as often as possible.
*   Balance our weight. When standing, this means distributing your weight evenly over both legs. When sitting, avoid crossing your legs, and avoid leaning to the left or right.

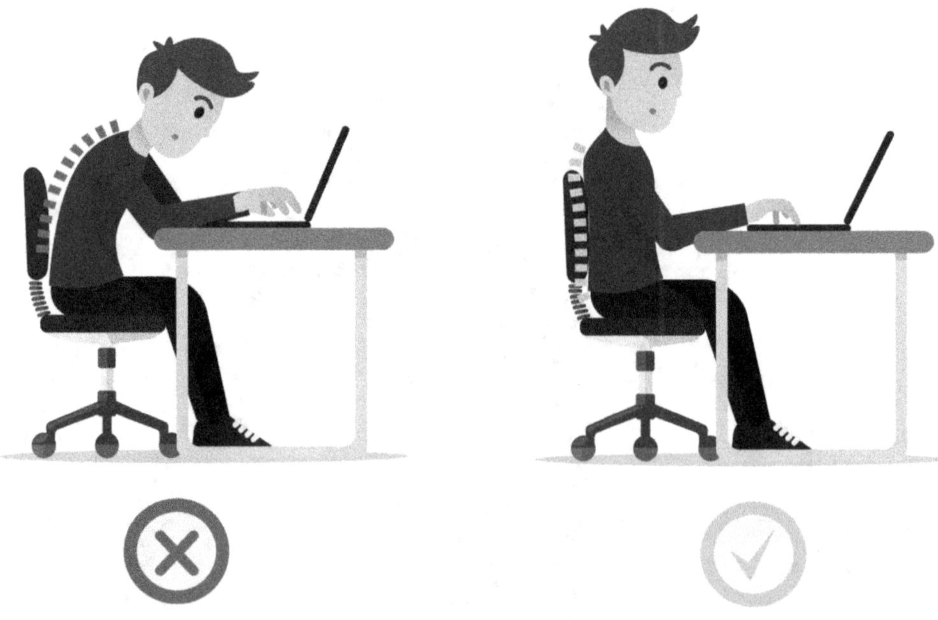

It should also be noted that bad posture can have consequences for our health, and can cause, among other things:
- Headaches.
- Lower back, back or neck pain.
- Reduced lung capacity.
- Digestive problems.
- Impaired blood circulation.

Of course, posture problems don't affect everyone. Some of us may have exemplary posture. However, if we're aiming for a flat stomach, we're going to need to do a few exercises to tone up our abdominal muscles.

Our back muscles are antagonistic to our abdominal muscles, and vice versa.
This means that when our abdominal muscles contract, the dorsal muscles (antagonistic muscles) stretch. Conversely, when the dorsal muscles contract, our abdominal muscles become the antagonist muscles and stretch in turn.

To avoid creating an imbalance, we therefore need to tone both the abdominal and back muscles.

It's time to put on our gym suit!

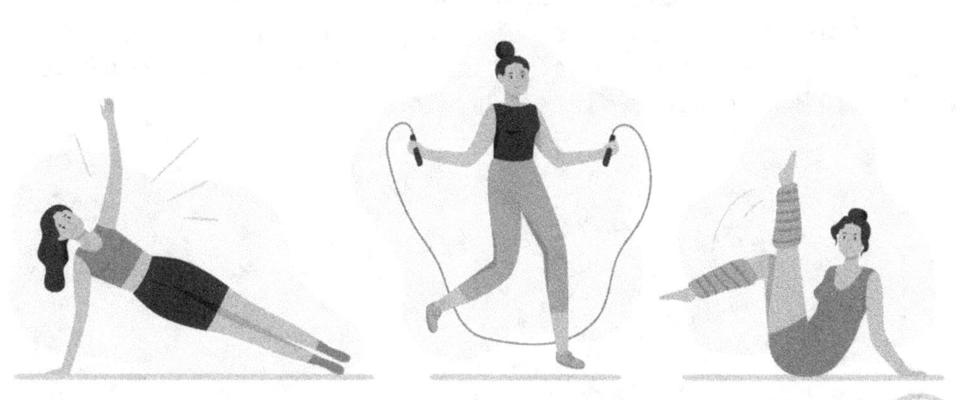

HOW TO TONE STOMACH AND BACK

There are a multitude of exercises for building and toning abdominal and back muscles.

We'll take a look at a few of them in the following pages. These are basic, simple exercises that anyone can do. No equipment is required, apart from a gym or yoga mat.

It is possible to create more complete sessions, for example with equipment (weights, elastics) or with other exercises. In this case, the Internet is our friend! There are lots of sites with very well-done instructional videos.

This section is aimed primarily at people with little or no physical activity, and who lack abdominal tone. However, those who already practice a sport of some kind will find information to help them improve their training or complete their sessions.

The exercises are divided into 5 categories: Transverse, obliques, rectus abdominis, back stretching and back muscles.

As a reminder, working the abdominal muscles helps to tone the waistline.

We'll be focusing primarily on the transverse abdominis muscle, which plays a fundamental role in maintaining a flat stomach. This will better support our viscera, reduce the circumference of our belly, and thus contribute to our ultimate goal (a flat stomach).

Working on the back muscles will have a complementary action, promoting better body support and improving posture.

For effective results, we'll perform at least three exercises for the transversus abdominis, one exercise for the obliques, one exercise for the rectus abdominis, and one exercise for the dorsi. Finally, I'd also advise you to do a back-stretching exercise, especially if you have postural problems or back tension.

Ideally, we'll perform a series of exercises. We'll perform one series, linking together all the exercises we've chosen, one after the other, then take a 2 to 3-minute rest. Then we'll do a second set, followed by a third (again, with a rest between each set).

For some exercises, we need to hold a position for as long as possible. Ideally, this is between 1 and 2 minutes, but for beginners, 30 seconds is a good target.

A session lasts about 20 to 30 minutes. We'll do at least one session every other day, and if we can, one session a day.

For beginners, we'll observe the following guidelines:
- Always wear suitable clothing (i.e. sportswear).
- Exercise in a calm, temperate environment.
- Make controlled, unhurried movements.
- Do not eat less than one hour before training.
- Hydrate regularly, without excess.

TRANSVERSE

PLANK

Position yourself as shown, elbows on the floor. Core your abdominal muscles and keep your back straight. Hold this position for as long as possible.

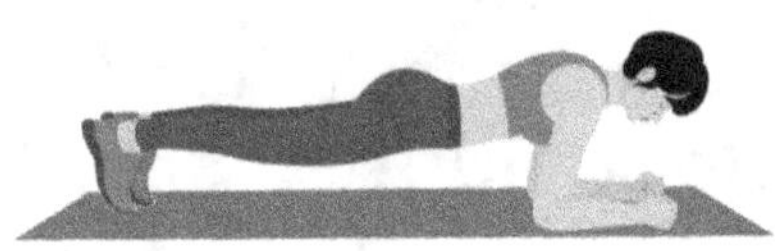

If your shoulders are tense, perform this exercise with your hands on the floor and your arms straight.

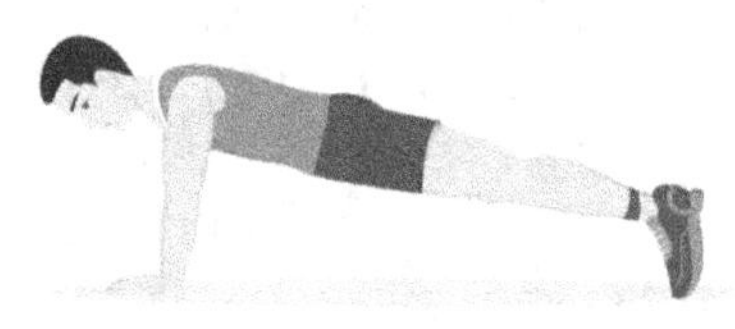

SIDE PLANK

Lie on your side, resting on your elbow. The opposite elbow points skyward. Raise your hips. Your body should be straight (head, hips and feet aligned). Hold the position, then switch sides. It's important to hold the position for the same amount of time on each side.

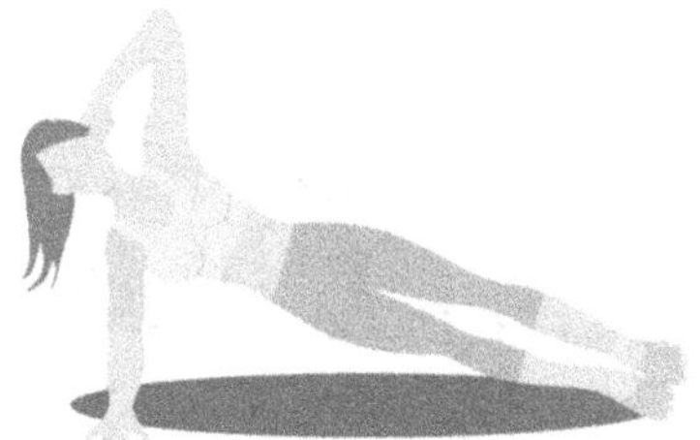

LEG RAISES

Lie on your back, arms at your sides. Contract your abdominal muscles and slowly raise your legs as high as possible, keeping them straight. Lower them gently, keeping your abdominals contracted.
Do as many repetitions as you can.

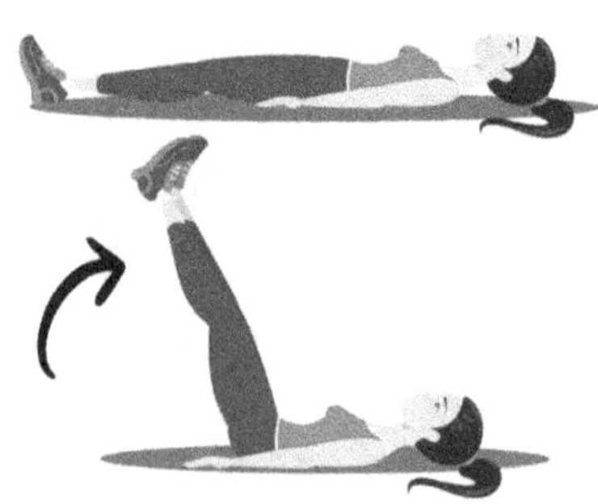

SHEATHING ON A CHAIR

Sit in a chair, leaning back slightly. Your back should be straight and resting on the backrest. Place your hands as shown. Contract your abdominal muscles and straighten your legs horizontally. Hold for as long as possible.

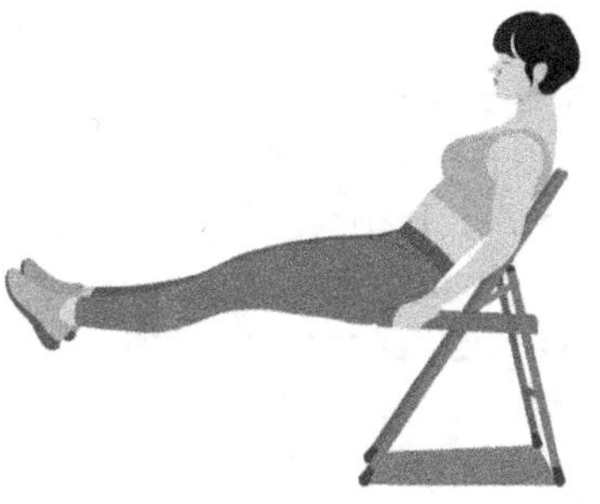

SCISSORS

Lie on your back, arms at your sides, head slightly raised. Keep your legs straight throughout the exercise. Contract your abdominal muscles and lift your feet off the floor. Raise one leg to about 35° (as shown), then lower it while raising the other leg. Keep up a steady rhythm and do as many repetitions as possible.

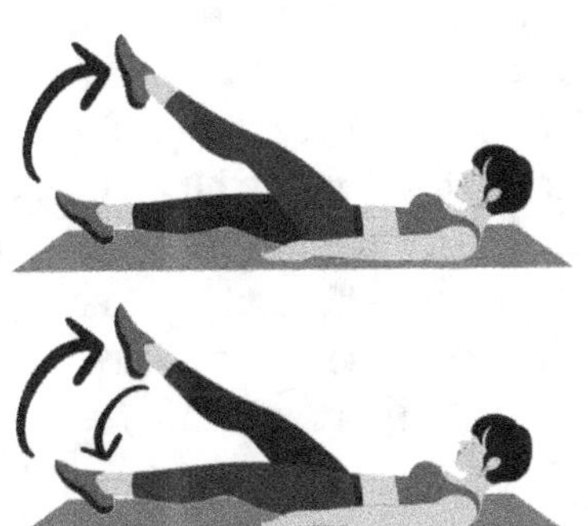

STOMACH VACUUM

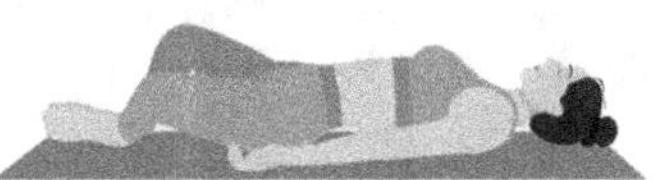

Lie on your back and exhale completely, contracting your abdominal muscles. Hold your breath and pull your stomach in as far as it will go, as if you wanted your navel to touch your spine. Hold the contraction for a few seconds, then release. Repeat at least 10 times.

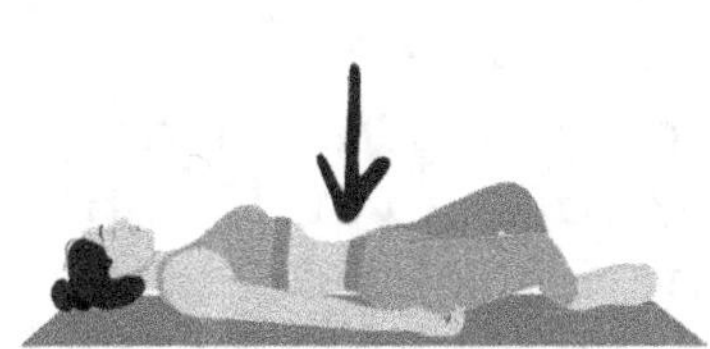

OBLIQUES

SIDE PLANKS WITH ROTATION

Get into a side plank position. Then lower your elbow towards your hand (on the floor), while rolling up your torso. Return to the starting position and repeat as many times as possible. Switch sides and do the same number of repetitions.

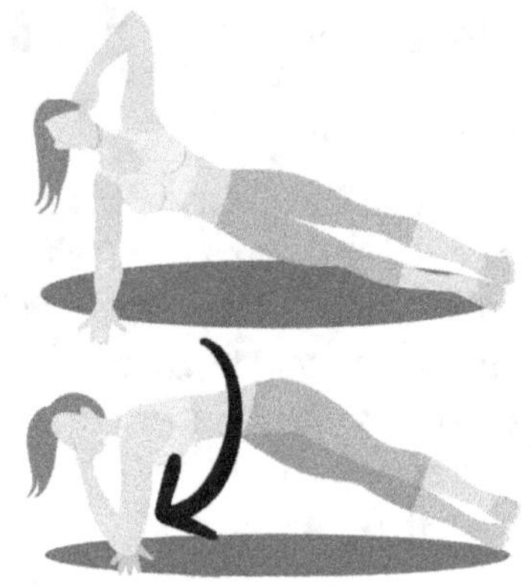

OBLIQUE CRUNCHES

Lie on your back, hands at ear level. Lift your heels slightly off the floor. Lift your upper back and bring one knee towards your chest, twisting so that the opposite knee and elbow touch. Return to the starting position and alternate movements (left knee/right elbow, and vice versa).

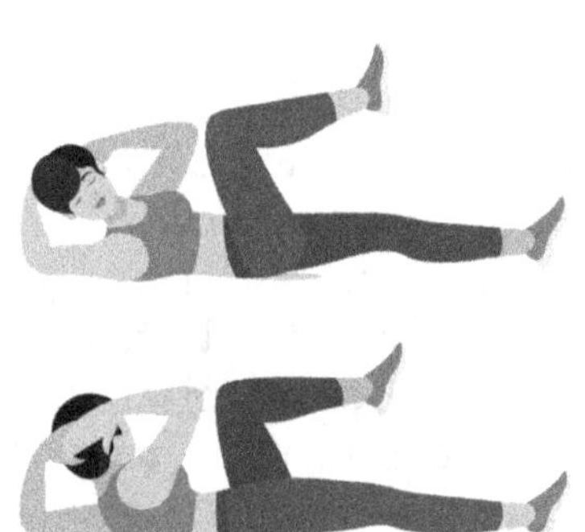

CROSS BODY MOUNTAIN CLIMBER

Place yourself in a plank position, leaning on your hands with your legs straight. Bring your right knee towards your left elbow, then return to the starting position. Then bring your left knee towards your right elbow. Do as many repetitions as possible, keeping a steady rhythm.

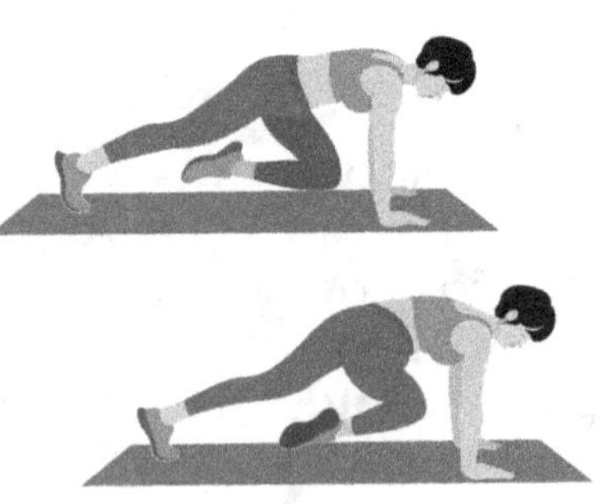

PLANK TWIST

Get into a plank position, resting on your elbows. Core your abdominal muscles and keep your back straight. Slowly rotate your hips to one side, then the other, and so on.
Do as many repetitions as you can.

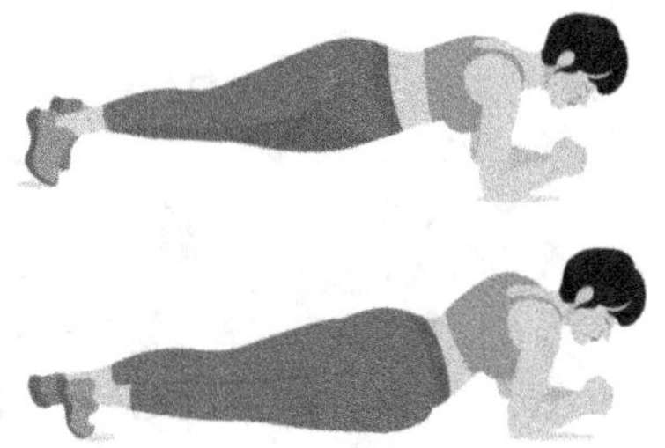

RUSSIAN TWISTS

Sit on the floor and tilt your back slightly backwards. Extend your arms forward, join your hands and raise your feet slightly. Rotate your torso so that your hands pass from one side to the other of your knees. Repeat for as long as possible.
If the exercise is too difficult, place your feet on the floor.

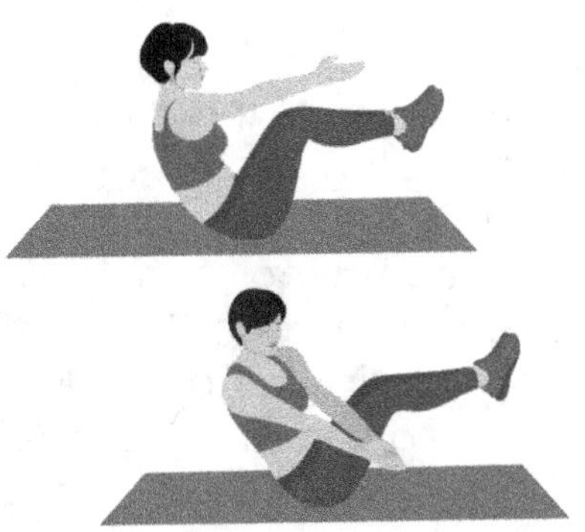

ANKLE TOUCHES

Lie on your back, bend your legs and lift your torso slightly off the floor. Extend your arms towards your ankles, then tilt your torso to the right to touch your right ankle. Return to the starting position, then do the same on the other side, and so on. Do as many repetitions as possible.

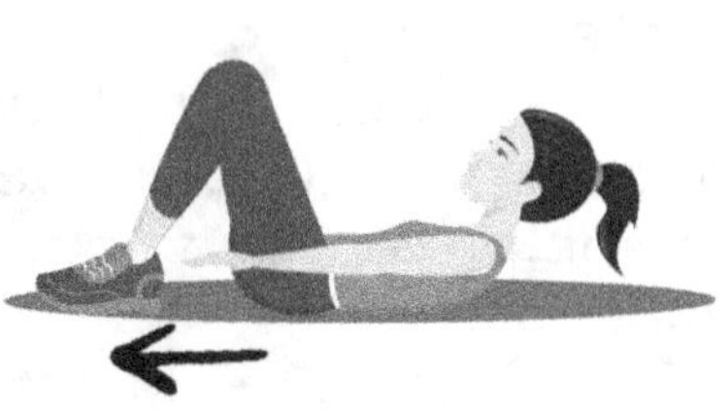

RECTUS ABDOMINIS

CRUNCHES

Lie on your back, legs bent and feet on the floor. Place your hands at ear level and lift your chest off the floor. Return to the starting position and repeat as many times as possible.

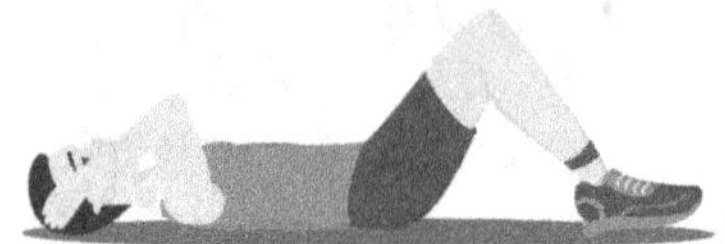

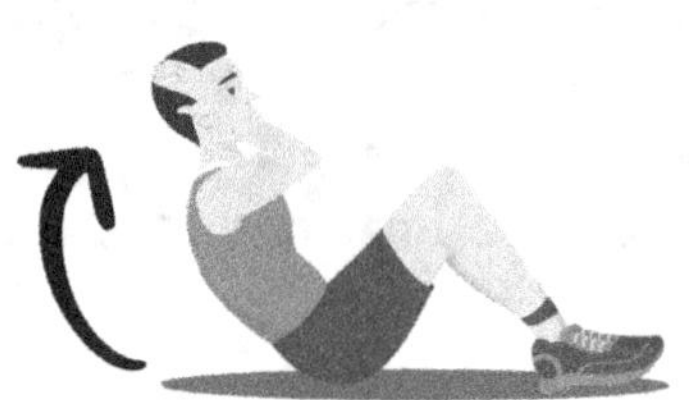

FEET-UP CRUNCHES

This is a variation on the above exercise.

The starting position is identical. Then lift your feet off the floor, and bring your knees slightly towards your chest with each lift. Do as many repetitions as possible.

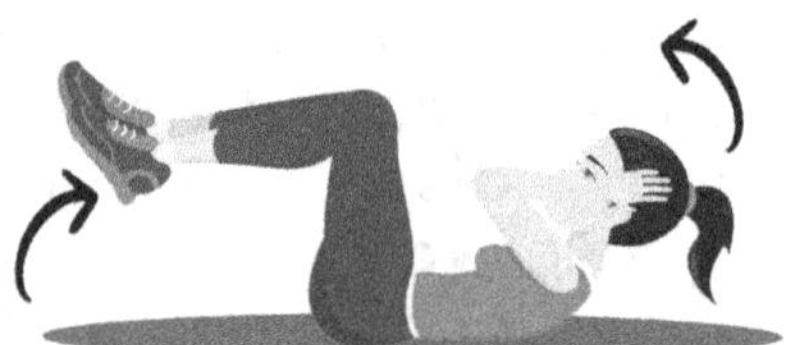

REVERSE CRUNCHES

Lie on your back and lift your feet off the floor, bending your legs at 90°. Position your arms at your sides. Bring your knees towards your face, contracting your abdominal muscles. Be careful not to help yourself too much with your arms.
Return to the starting position and repeat as many times as possible.

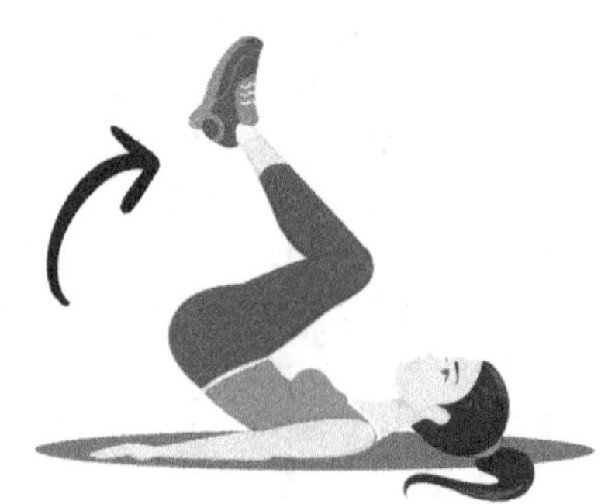

WALLET CRUNCHES

Lie on your back, legs straight, arms stretched behind your head and hands clasped.
 Contract your abdominal muscles and simultaneously lift your arms and legs, keeping them straight. Hold for 2-3 seconds, then return to the starting position. Repeat at least 10 times.

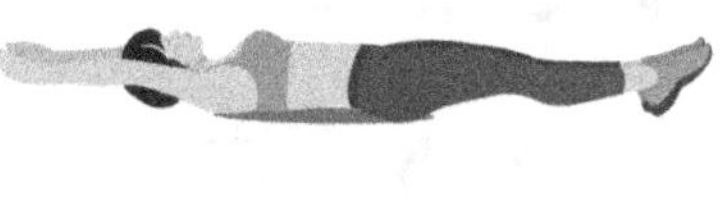

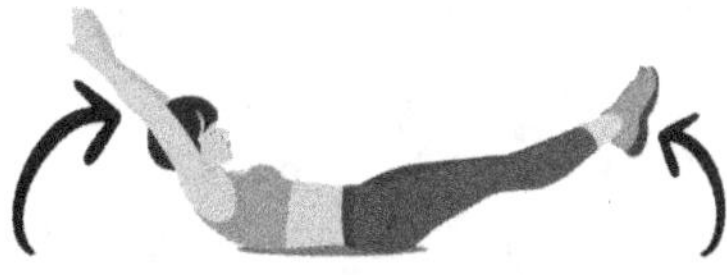

HOW TO STRETCH THE BACK

THE COW AND THE CAT

This exercise comes from yoga. Get down on all fours. Inhale, deepening the back and lifting the head. Exhale, tilting the pelvis down and rounding the spine. Bring your chin towards your chest and pull in your stomach. Repeat at least 10 times.

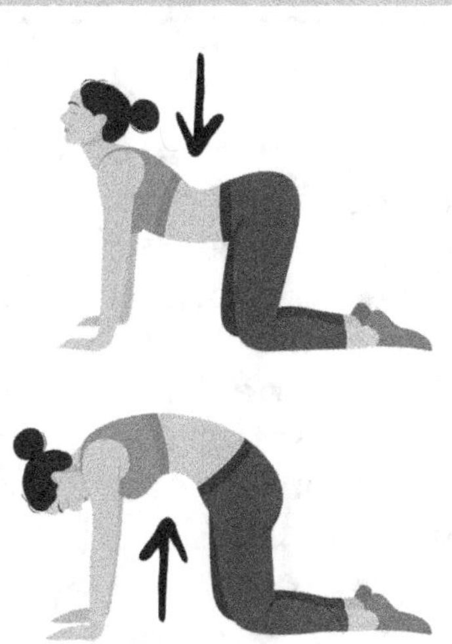

THE SPHINX AND THE COBRA

Another yoga exercise.
For the sphinx: Lie on your stomach. Position elbows under shoulders, legs together. Inhale, raising your upper body slightly, and exhale, releasing gently. You can also switch to the cobra position: as you inhale, straighten your arms, then rest your elbows on the floor as you exhale.

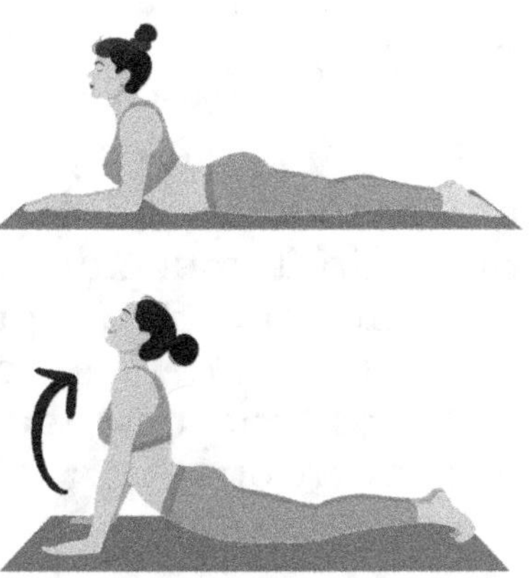

THE BACK

THE TWO-LEGGED TABLE

Get down on all fours, back straight, and sheath your abdominal muscles. Raise one arm and the opposite leg. Return to the starting position and reverse the movement.

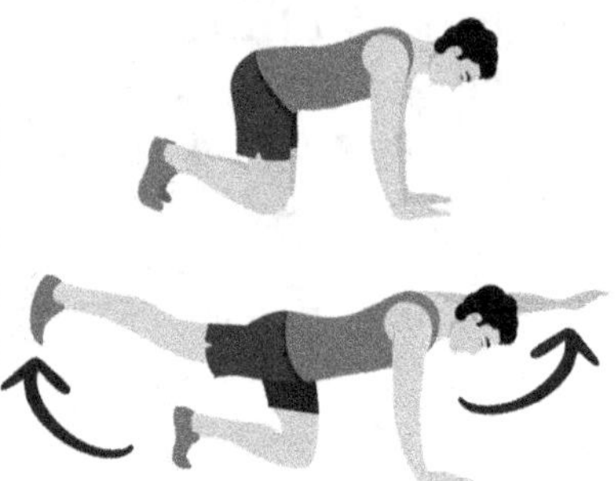

Do at least 10 repetitions on each side.

THE SWIMMER

Lie on your stomach. Extend your arms forward and spread your legs slightly. Raise your head and lift arms and legs slightly off the ground.
Raise one arm and the opposite leg. Return to the starting position and reverse the movement.
Do at least 10 repetitions on each side.

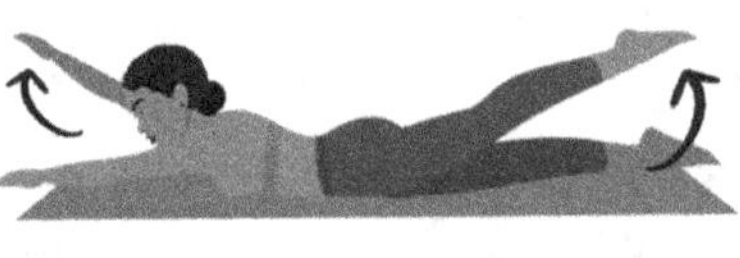

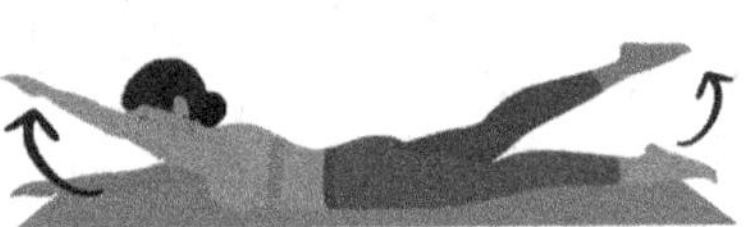

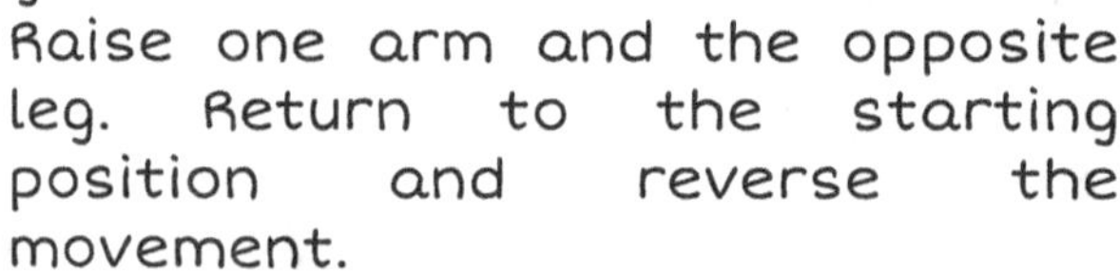

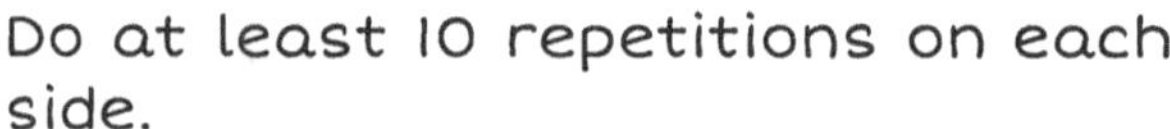

THE HIP TRUST

Lie on your back, arms at your sides and legs bent. Contract your abdominal muscles and lift your hips off the floor, pushing lightly on your heels. Hold for 2-3 seconds and release. Do at least 10 repetitions.

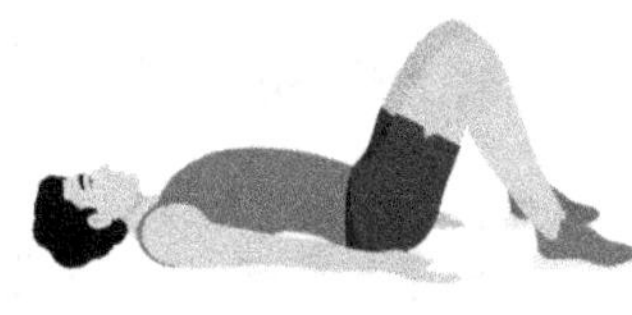

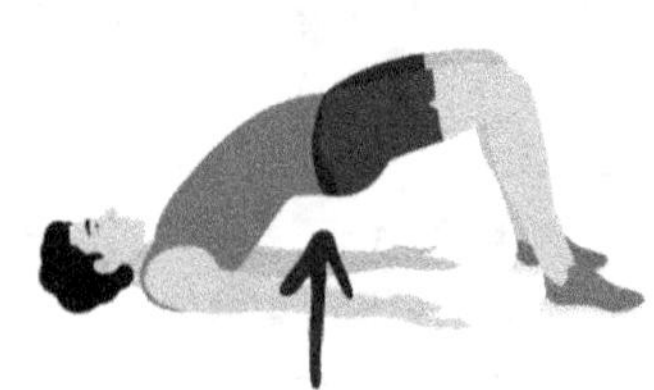

SQUATS

Stand with feet shoulder-width apart. Core your abdominal muscles.
Slowly lower yourself down, arms out, tilting your torso and keeping your back straight. Slowly pull yourself up, starting by raising your torso.
Do at least 10 repetitions.

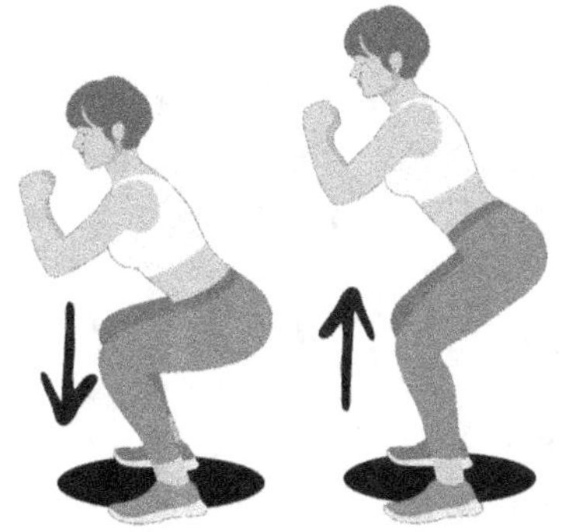

SUPERMAN

Lie on your stomach. Squeeze your legs together. Stretch your arms out in front of you.

Lift your legs and arms off the floor and hold for a few seconds. Release and repeat.
Do at least 10 repetitions.

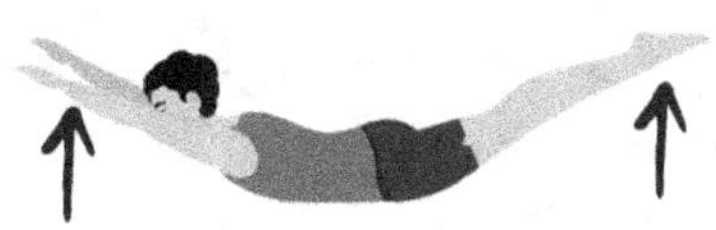

STRAIGHT-LEG DEADLIFT

Take a light weight in each hand (a dumbbell, a water bottle, etc.). Weights should be identical. Remain standing, and contract your abdominal muscles. Bend forward, keeping your back straight and your legs straight. Return to the starting position, concentrating on the contraction of the lower back muscles. Repeat at least 10 times.

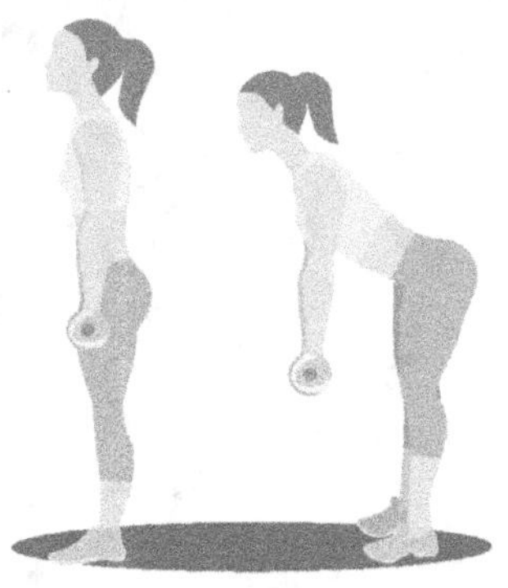

WORKOUT EXAMPLE

Here's an example of a program to set up, with a training session every two days MINIMUM for people with little or no physical activity.

FIRST SERIES

Plank
Objective: Hold position for at least 1 minute.
Leg raises
Goal: Hold position for at least 1 minute.
Vacuum stomach
Goal: Do at least 10 repetitions.
Ankle touches
Goal: Do at least 20 repetitions on each side.
Feet-up crunches
Goal: Do at least 30 reps.
Superman
Objective: Do at least 20 repetitions.
Cow and cat
Objective: Do at least 10 repetitions.

TAKE 3 MINUTES REST

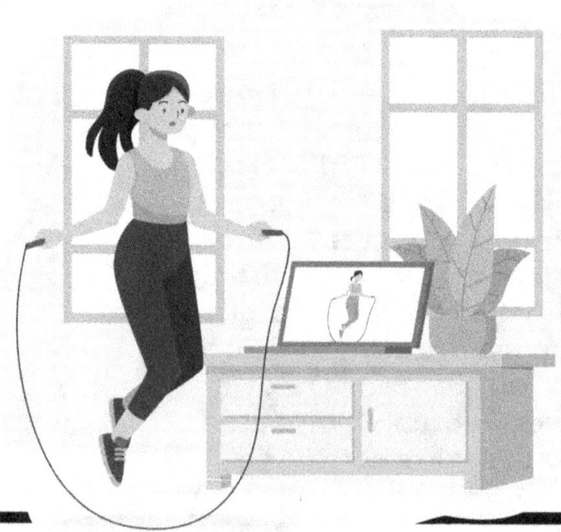

SECOND SERIES

Plank
Objective: Hold position for at least 1 minute.
Leg raises
Goal: Hold position for at least 1 minute.
Vacuum stomach
Goal: Do at least 10 repetitions.
Ankle touches
Goal: Do at least 20 repetitions on each side.
Feet-up crunches
Goal: Do at least 30 reps.
Superman
Objective: Do at least 20 repetitions.
Cow and cat
Objective: Do at least 10 repetitions.

TAKE 3 MINUTES REST

THIRD SERIES

Plank
Objective: Hold position for at least 1 minute.
Leg raises
Goal: Hold position for at least 1 minute.
Vacuum stomach
Goal: Do at least 10 repetitions.
Ankle touches
Goal: Do at least 20 repetitions on each side.
Feet-up crunches
Goal: Do at least 30 reps.
Superman
Objective: Do at least 20 repetitions.
Cow and cat
Objective: Do at least 10 repetitions.

HOW TO BURN FAT

Now we're going to take a look at sporting activity with a new objective in mind: burning fat.

As we have seen, fat accumulates when calorie intake exceeds energy requirements. We've learned to balance our diet, both qualitatively and quantitatively, and this can be enough to trigger weight loss.

For some of us, however, it may not be enough. Maybe our body fat is too high and our diet rebalancing isn't enough. Maybe we can't create enough of a caloric deficit to initiate significant weight loss.

This is where physical activity comes in.

The exercises we've just seen were designed to tone our abdominal and back muscles to achieve a flat stomach (by acting on the transverse muscle in particular) and to correct any poor posture. Although highly beneficial, these exercises require a relatively low caloric expenditure.

You can estimate that a session like the one described on the previous page will burn between 100 and 200 Kcal. Not a lot, especially if you do one every other day.

There are several mechanisms involved in burning fat through physical activity:
Depending on the type of exercise or sport, the body needs varying amounts of energy. If we are already in a caloric deficit, even a slight one, our body will have to draw on its reserves (i.e. fat).

Physical activity also has a stimulating effect on our metabolism. This is particularly true of cardiovascular activities (i.e. those that significantly increase our heart rate), which tend to speed up our metabolism, making it easier to burn fat.

Physical activity also helps to maintain and build muscle mass. Our muscles consume a lot of energy when we exercise, but they also consume energy at rest. In other words, the more muscular we are, the more calories our body will burn.

Last but not least, sporting activities contribute to the overall functioning of our body, and have a beneficial influence on our hormonal balance. What's more, it's an excellent way of combating stress and getting a good night's sleep.

That's why it's so important to take part in regular sporting activities, whether in a club or on your own at home.

But what if we can't do sport? There are plenty of other, non-sporting activities that burn energy (and therefore calories).

Bowling, for example, can burn up to 250 Kcal in an hour. Gardening can burn up to 400 Kcal/hour. Playing music can burn up to 350 Kcal, as can fishing (non-static, i.e. walking along a river).

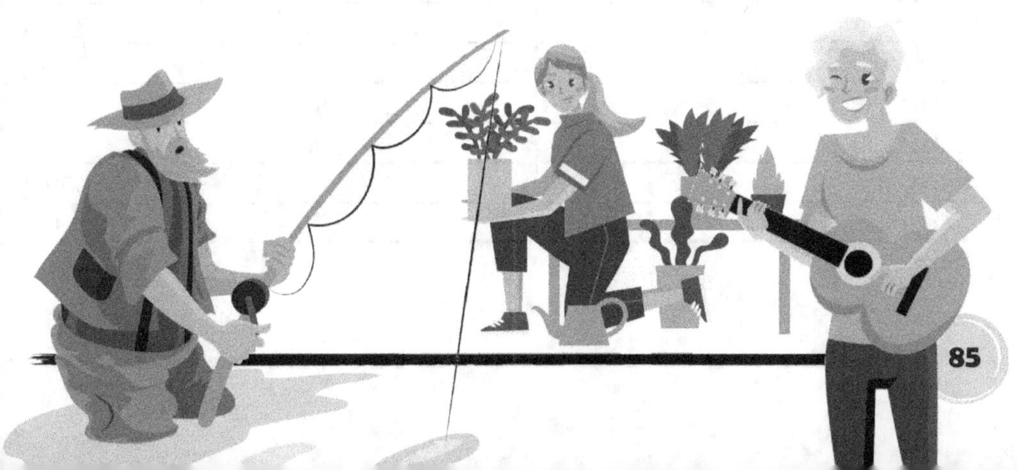

LIST OF SPORTS ACTIVITIES

Here's a list of common sporting activities, classified according to the energy expenditure they generate.

These estimates may vary according to intensity, but also to muscle mass, age, sex... That's why there is a low estimate and a high estimate.

The low estimate corresponds to exercise at a moderate pace, and the high estimate to exercise at a steady pace.

Depending on our objectives (fat loss), our possibilities and our preferences, let's try to practice one of these activities at least twice a week (and more often if possible).

Practising one (or more) of these activities will accelerate our fat loss and contribute to our general well-being.

SPORT / ACTIVITY	ENERGY EXPENDITURE (in Kcal / hour)	
	LOW ESTIMATE	HIGH ESTIMATE
Billards	120	180
Archery	150	250
Bowling	150	250
Golf	200	350
Surfing	250	350
Baseball	250	350
Curling	200	350
Walking	250	400
Scuba diving	300	400
Aquagym	300	400
Swimming (leisure)	300	400

SPORT / ACTIVITY	ENERGY EXPENDITURE (in Kcal / hour)	
	LOW ESTIMATE	HIGH ESTIMATE
Badminton	350	450
Table tennis	350	450
Kayak	400	500
Pilates	350	500
Bodybuilding	250	500
Weightlifting	250	500
Dance	250	500
Fencing	350	500
Volleyball	250	500
Skateboarding	300	500
Swimming (sport)	400	600
Tennis	400	600
Basketball	500	600
Downhill skiing	450	600
Horseback riding	450	600
Aerobics / Gymnastics	350	600
Running	550	700
Soccer	600	700
Cross country skiing	550	700
Climbing	600	700
Rowing	450	700
Boxing	600	700
American football / rugby	600	700
Aquabike	500	700
Cricket / Lacrosse	400	700
Polo	450	700
Ice skating	450	850
Squash	700	850
Skipping rope	700	850
Martial arts	700	850
Water polo	600	900
Biking	400	1000

A HEALTHY BODY

As we've just seen, physical activity is really important for our health.

Exercises targeting the abdominal and back muscles help firm up the stomach and promote better posture.

Practising another physical activity increases energy expenditure, helping to create a calorie deficit.

Let's take the example of a person who does little physical activity, and whose energy requirements are 2000 Kcal, or 14,000 Kcal per week.

By improving their diet, this person will create a caloric deficit of 200 Kcal per day, or 1400 Kcal per week.

If this person starts cycling at a moderate pace (at around 500 Kcal/hour), for 3 hours a week, they will increase their energy expenditure by 1500 Kcal/week.

Combined with a balanced diet, the caloric deficit will be almost 3000 Kcal per week, i.e. more than 21% of requirements.

Of course, if we're not really sporty, it's hard to find the motivation to get on a bike or join a fitness club.

But we mustn't lose sight of our goal. Our belly won't magically become flat. Isn't our well-being worth 2 or 3 hours of sport a week?

Throughout this book, we've seen that diet and physical activity are of vital importance in our quest for a flat stomach.

But certain hormonal mechanisms can affect the achievement of our goals, and sometimes wreck our efforts.

Apart from any health problems, it's mainly sleep disorders and stress that can lead to dysfunctions at this level.

So we're going to look at these phenomena, understand them and provide simple solutions to these problems.

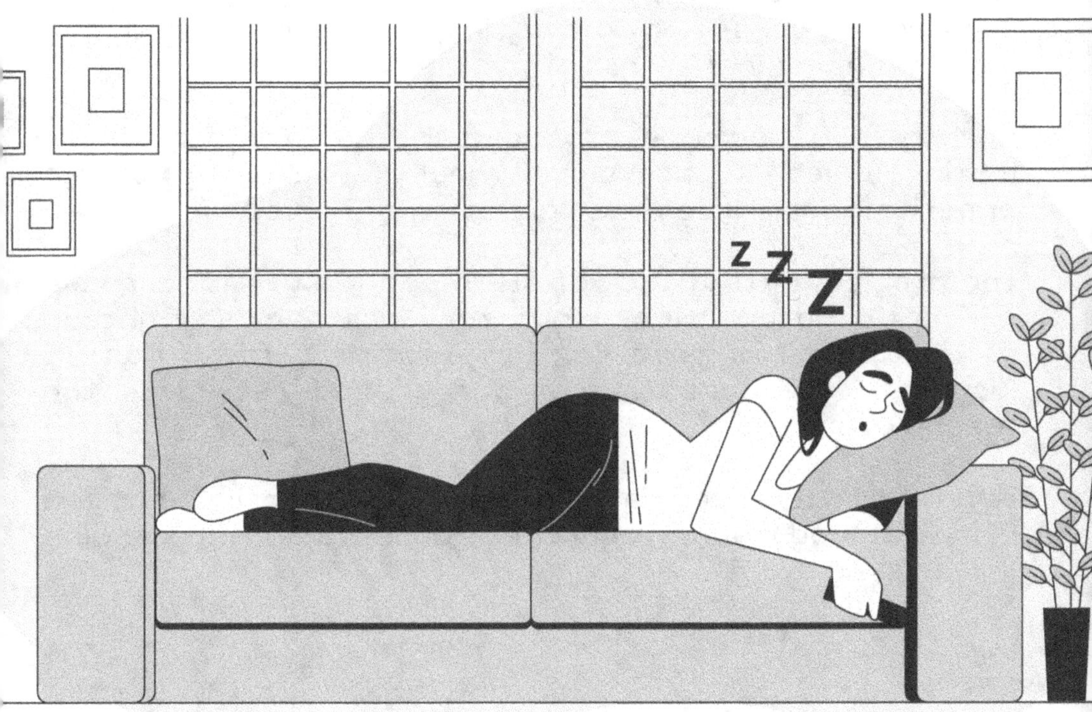

SLEEP

Sleep plays a crucial role in the proper functioning of our metabolism.

We've all noticed that a lack of sleep has an impact on our concentration, mood and physical energy.

But what few people know is that lack of sleep has a major influence on the accumulation of fat in our bodies.

Let's see how it all works.

Lack of sleep influences the production of two hormones: leptin and ghrelin.

Leptin is a hormone produced in adipose tissue (i.e. fat). It plays an important role in regulating appetite, since it creates a sensation of satiety. In other words, it suppresses hunger.

Ghrelin is a hormone produced in the stomach. Unlike leptin, which suppresses hunger, ghrelin stimulates appetite and reduces the sensation of satiety.

The problem is that lack of sleep can lead to a decrease in leptin production and an increase in ghrelin production. This has a devastating effect, as it increases the sensation of hunger and decreases the feeling of satiety.

It should also be noted that sleep deprivation can disrupt blood sugar regulation, once again encouraging fat accumulation.

All this becomes a vicious circle: lack of sleep increases our appetite, which is likely to encourage overeating (and thus increase calorie intake). Since we don't sleep well, we're going to feel tired. This physical and mental fatigue will disrupt our daily lives. We won't have the energy or motivation to be physically active, and perhaps we won't have the courage to cook healthy meals. The end result will be further weight gain, and even greater demotivation.

So we mustn't neglect the quality of our sleep.

Here are a few tips to help you sleep better:
- Go to bed and get up at the same time every day, to regulate our rhythm.
- Avoid stimulants (coffee, alcohol, tobacco) at least 4 hours before bedtime.
- Avoid exposure to screens at least one hour before bedtime. Blue light stimulates the retina and disrupts our biological clock.
- Keep our bedroom temperature between 16 and 20°C (60/68°F), and sleep without any light sources.
- Avoid heavy meals in the evening.

It's also important to remember that physical activity helps you fall asleep and improves sleep quality.

Certain activities, such as reading or listening to music, can also help you relax before going to sleep.

Finally, if sleep problems persist, you should consult a doctor for advice and appropriate solutions.

Ideally, we should be getting at least 7 to 8 hours' sleep a night.

STRESS

Like sleep, stress has an influence on our weight gain, and therefore our ability to eliminate fat.

Being stressed from time to time is perfectly normal, but when this stress becomes regular, or even permanent, it upsets our metabolism.

When we are in a stressful situation, our body (and more specifically our adrenal glands) secretes cortisol, also known as the stress hormone. The main role of this hormone is to give us a quick energy boost in situations where we need to flee or fight, for example.

Cortisol promotes the production of glucose (sugar) and the release of fat, to provide our muscles with rapid energy. But when cortisol levels regularly become too high, our body will seek to renew fat stocks. As a result, we'll crave food (often sweet foods), and tend to store fat. Excess cortisol also has the effect of degrading muscle mass, which in turn reduces our energy expenditure.

Chronic stress will also affect our daily lives: loss or increase in appetite, increase in tobacco or alcohol consumption, reduced energy, loss of motivation, disrupted sleep cycle...

It's not always easy to eliminate sources of stress, but we do need to take action if we are to achieve our goals.

For example, physical activity helps reduce cortisol levels, especially in the morning (cortisol production is at its highest after waking up).

Yoga and meditation are also highly beneficial. Recent studies by the University of California have shown that daily yoga practice significantly reduces cortisol levels after 3 months.

It's also important to understand that if we limit excessively rich foods (sugar and fat), we also limit cortisol peaks.

Quality sleep also helps reduce stress.

Finally, the effects of chronic stress are generally very harmful, and can lead to heart or digestive problems, muscular tension or emotional disorders...

Let's not let stress take over our lives.

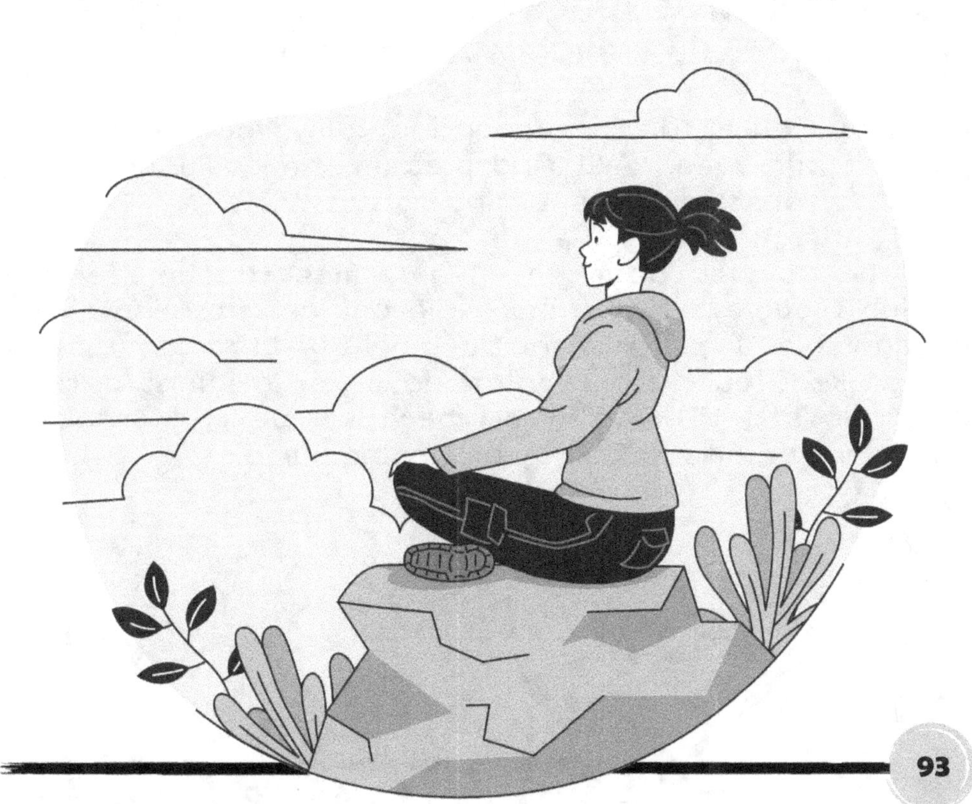

IN CONCLUSION

We've come to the end of this book.

We've discovered a lot!

We've understood the mechanisms that led us to gain fat and have a (slightly, very) rounded belly.

We know how to adopt a healthy, balanced diet, and how to set up a calorie deficit to allow the body to draw on its reserves.

We've discovered the importance of physical activity for our health, and we know which exercises to do to tone our abdominal muscles, correct our posture, or increase our energy expenditure.

Now we have all the knowledge we need to take effective long-term action. There's no reason to fail, no excuse to give up.

Our new habits (dietary, sporting) will gradually become part of our lives. We'll find pleasure in cooking healthy meals, or practicing a sporting activity.

We'll be able to adapt our new rules to our lifestyle. Having trouble maintaining a dietary deficit? Who cares, we can take up a sport that will help us burn fat (as long as we keep our intake balanced or at a slight deficit). Can't do sport? No matter, because we can create a sufficient caloric deficit by balancing our diet.

If we are truly committed to our well-being and to achieving our goals, we will succeed.

And once we've achieved our goal?

Well, that's simple... We'll maintain a healthy diet and, if possible, continue to exercise. But once we've reached our goal, we'll need to stabilize our calorie intake, since we no longer need to create a deficit.

To do this, we'll need to calculate our TDEE again (based on our new energy expenditure). We can then increase our intake slightly, so that it equals our TDEE. This way, we won't lose any more body fat, but we won't accumulate any either.

Let's continue to take care of ourselves, and be proud of every effort, every result... And smile at our mirror every time we walk past.

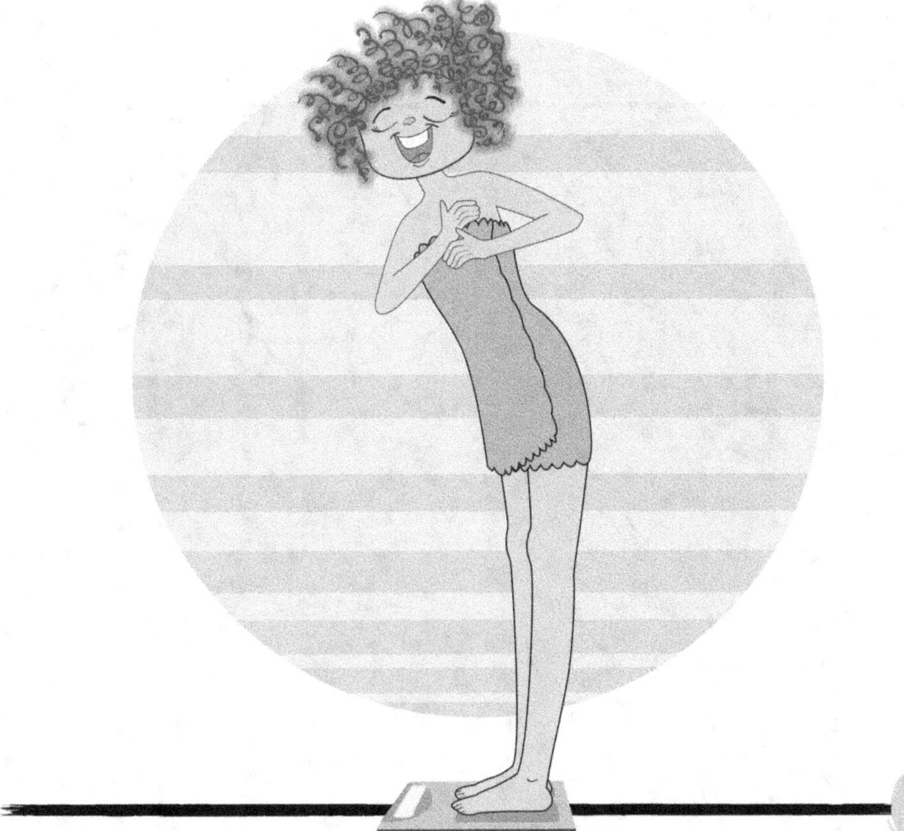

APPENDIX

This appendix contains :

- Nutrition tables showing the calorie and macronutrient content of the most common foods.

- The daily calorie intake calculation sheet, in duplicate. Feel free to reproduce or photocopy.

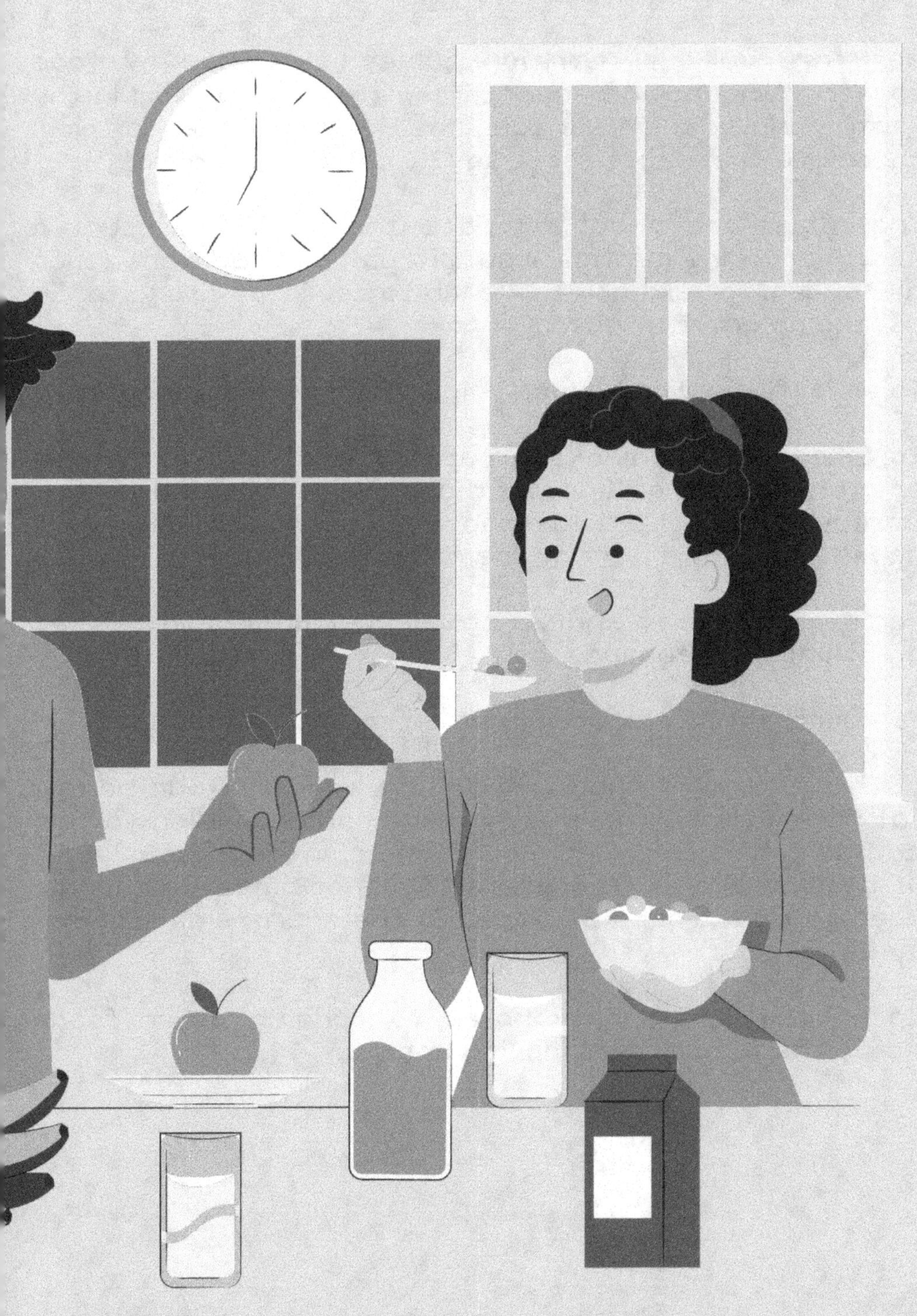

NUTRITION TABLES

Here are various nutrition tables, classified by food category. Weights and quantities refer to products in the form in which they are consumed. For example, for rice, these are the values for 100g (3.5 Oz) of cooked rice.

The values are global estimates, taking into account a healthy cooking method, and without any additions (such as sauces, for example). In each table, foods are listed in ascending order of energy intake.

To simplify reading, values below 0.5 have been ignored.

For meats (excluding charcuterie) and fish, estimates are based on grilling methods, with no added fat. Moreover, these are average values, which may vary depending on the part of the animal.

For starchy foods and vegetables, estimates are based on boiling or steaming.

For fruit, estimates are based on raw products.

If the cooking method is modified, with the addition of fat for example, the energy value corresponding to this addition must be added. For example, in the case of a rib of beef cooked in 50 grams (1.75 Oz) of butter, we would need to add around 380 Kcal to the energy value of our meat.

Each table has empty boxes for adding other foods according to our consumption habits.

MEATS

FOOD for 100 g (3.5 Oz)	ENERGY Kcal	PROTEINS grams	CARBS grams	FATS grams
Deer / Roe deer	115	20	0	4
Rabbit	130	21	0	5
Turkey	135	30	0	1,5
Chicken	140	29	0	3
Lamb / Mutton	145	25	0	5
Wild boar	145	20	0	7
Ostrich	150	22	0	7
Horse	150	24	0	6
Eggs	150	14	0	10
Guinea fowl	155	23	0	7
Game birds	155	30	0	4
Offal	155	25	0	6
Pork	165	25	0	7
Beef	185	26	0	9
Duck	340	22	0	28

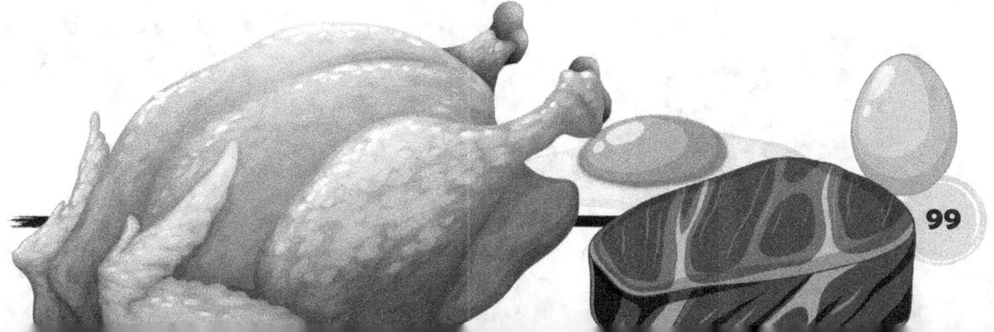

COLD CUTS / CHARCUTERIE

FOOD for 100 g (3.5 Oz)	ENERGY Kcal	PROTEINS grams	CARBS grams	FATS grams
Bacon	115	23	0	2,5
Ham	120	21	0	4
Beef jerky	200	37	1	5
Cured ham	220	21	0	15
Black pudding	255	14	2	21
Pâté	290	14	2	25
Sausage	335	19	8	25
Salami	340	25	2	26
Dry sausage	400	22	2	34
Rillettes	420	14	1	40
Chorizo	450	22	2	40

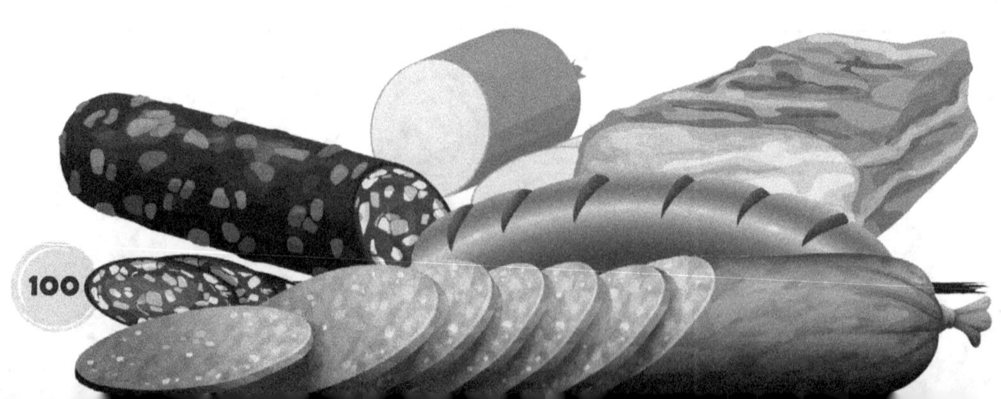

FISH AND SEAFOOD

	FOOD for 100 g (3.5 Oz)	ENERGY Kcal	PROTEINS grams	CARBS grams	FATS grams
Fatty fish	Tuna	150	26	0	5
	Trout	170	22	0	9
	Eel	180	18	0	12
	Salmon	200	21	0	13
	Sardines	200	25	0	11
	Herring	210	19	0	15
	Mackerel	250	20	0	19
Lean fish	Skate	90	20	0	1
	Sea bass	95	20	0	2
	Pollock	95	20	0	2
	Halibut	100	20	0	2
	Pike	105	20	0	3
	Cod	105	22	0	2
	Sea bream	110	23	0	2
	Carp	115	20	0	4
Shellfish / Crustaceans	Oysters	70	8	6	1,5
	Squid	80	16	0	1,5
	Octopus	80	17	0	1,5
	Mussels	85	12	4	2
	Lobster	95	19	0	2
	Shrimps	100	20	0	2
	Scallops	105	15	2	4
	Crab	135	20	0	6

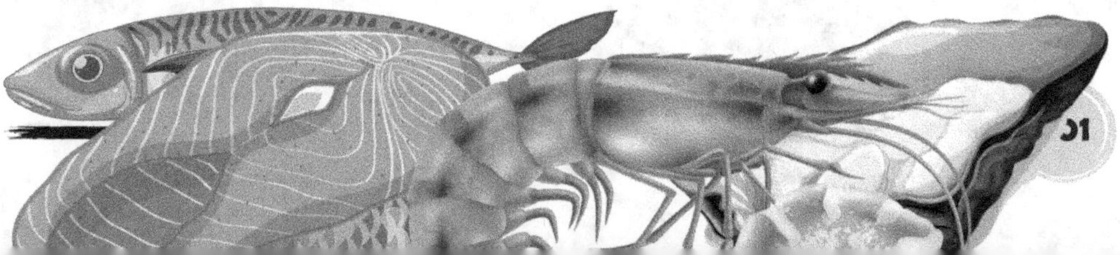

STARCHY FOOD

FOOD for 100 g (3.5 Oz)	ENERGY Kcal	PROTEINS grams	CARBS grams	FATS grams
Oats	70	2,5	12	1,5
Sweet potatoes	85	1,5	20	0
Potatoes	90	2	20	0
Corn	100	3	18	1,5
Wheat semolina	110	4	24	0
Kidney beans	115	8	14	3
Quinoa	120	4	21	2
Lentils	120	8	17	2
Chestnuts	120	2	24	1,5
Wheat, spelt	120	3,5	24	1
White / wholemeal rice	125	2,5	29	0
Pasta	130	6	25	1
Wholemeal bread	250	8	43	5
White bread	280	8	49	6

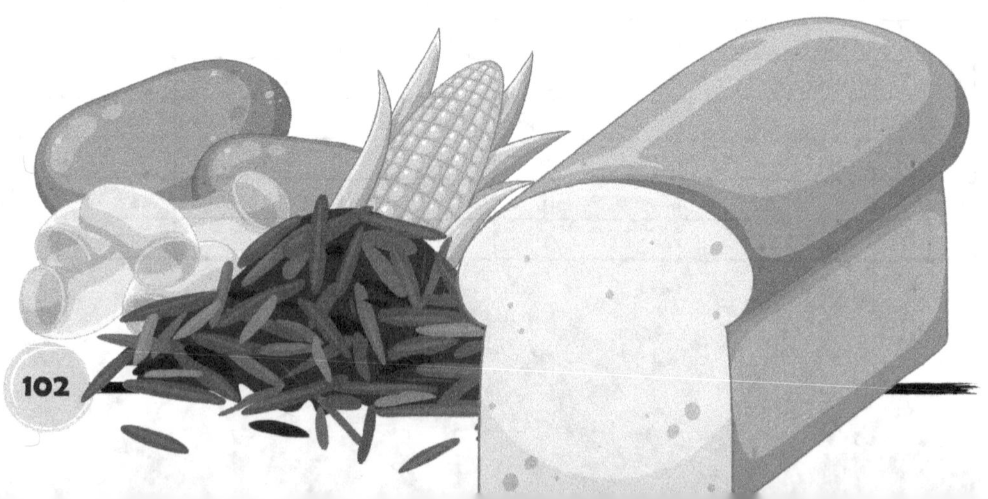

VEGETABLES

FOOD for 100 g (3.5 Oz)	ENERGY Kcal	PROTEINS grams	CARBS grams	FATS grams
Lettuce	12	1,5	1,5	0
Radish	15	0	3,5	0
Endive	18	1	3,5	0
Zucchini	20	1	4	0
Tomato	20	1	4	0
Asparagus	20	2	3	0
Spinach	25	2	4	0
Mushrooms	25	3	3	0
Leek	25	2	4	0
Eggplant	28	1	6	0
Cabbage / Cauliflower	28	2	5	0
Pumpkin	28	1	6	0
Green beans	30	1	7	0
Turnip	30	1	6,5	0
Broccoli	35	3	6	0
Peppers	40	1	9	0
Onion	40	1,5	8	0
Carrot	45	1	10	0
Squash / Butternut	45	1	11	0
Beet	45	2	9	0
Artichoke	50	2	11	0
Pea	75	5	14	0
Garlic	115	8	21	0
Avocado	160	2	9	13

DAIRY PRODUCTS

FOOD for 100 g (3.5 Oz)	ENERGY Kcal	PROTEINS grams	CARBS grams	FATS grams
Skimmed milk	35	4	5	0
Whole milk	60	3	5	3
Goat cheese	270	10	1	25
Mozzarella	290	30	2	18
Camembert	305	20	0	25
Roquefort	370	21	2	31
Emmental	390	28	2	30
Cheddar	400	25	0	33
Butter	770	1	0	85

FOOD for 100 g (3.5 Oz)	ENERGY Kcal	PROTEINS grams	CARBS grams	FATS grams
0% cottage cheese	35	5	4	0
sugar-free yogurt	60	4	5	3
Sweetened yogurt	75	4	12	1
Fruit yogurt	80	4	13	1,5
20% cottage cheese	105	6	5	7
Dessert cream	135	2	20	5

DESSERTS AND CAKES

FOOD for 100 g (3.5 Oz)	ENERGY Kcal	PROTEINS grams	CARBS grams	FATS grams
Frozen sorbet	105	2	24	0
Ice cream	210	3	25	11
Apple pie	240	1,5	35	10
Cream puff	250	3,5	25	15
Waffle	295	6	45	10
Tiramisu	310	4,5	23	22
Cheesecake	330	6	23	24
strawberry cake	330	4	24	24
Sugar crepe	350	5	70	6
Chocolate cakes	385	6	50	18
Cream cakes	400	5	45	22
Viennese pastries	405	7	45	22
Doughnut	460	7	45	28
Brownie	485	5	60	25
Cookie	500	6	62	26

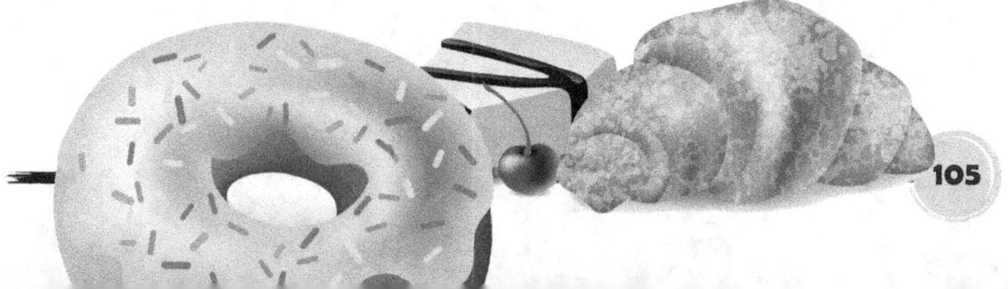

FRUITS

FOOD for 100 g (3.5 Oz)	ENERGY Kcal	PROTEINS grams	CARBS grams	FATS grams
Lemon	25	1	5	0
Watermelon	30	1	7	0
Strawberries	35	1	7,5	0
Melon	35	1	8	0
Orange	40	1	9	0
Peach	40	1	9	0
Apricot	40	1	9	0
Papaya	45	1	11	0
Apple	50	0	14	0
Cherries	50	1	12	0
Plum	50	1	11	0
Pineapple	55	1	13	0
Pear	60	0	15	0
Raspberry	60	1,5	12	0,5
Fig	60	1,5	13	0
Kiwi	65	1	15	0
Mango	65	1	15	0
Blackcurrant	70	1	17	0
Grapes	75	1	18	0
Pomegranate	85	2	19	0
Banana	90	1	22	0
Dried dates	260	3	62	0
Coconuts	350	3,5	3,5	35

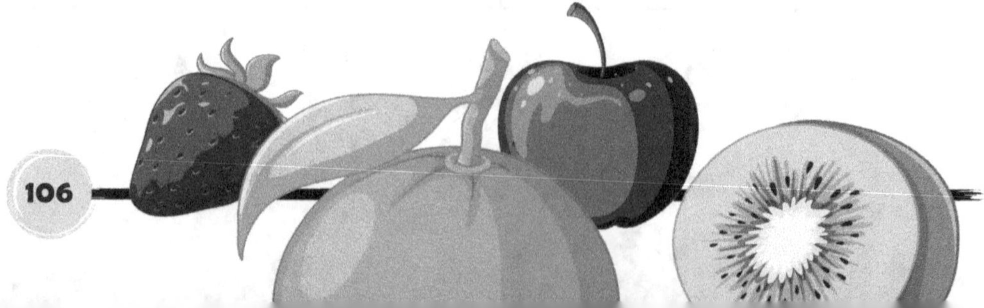

DRINKS

FOOD for 100 g (3.5 Oz)	ENERGY Kcal	PROTEINS grams	CARBS grams	FATS grams
Water	0	0	0	0
Sugar-free tea	1	0	0	0
Sugar-free coffee	2	0,5	0	0
Almond milk	15	0,5	0,5	1
Beer	30	0	2,5	0
Soy milk	33	3,5	1,5	1,5
Fruit juices	42	0,5	10	0
Soda / Lemonade	45	0	11	0
Energy drink	45	0	11	0
Champagne	80	0	2,5	0
Wine	82	0	2,5	0
Coconut milk	235	2	5	23

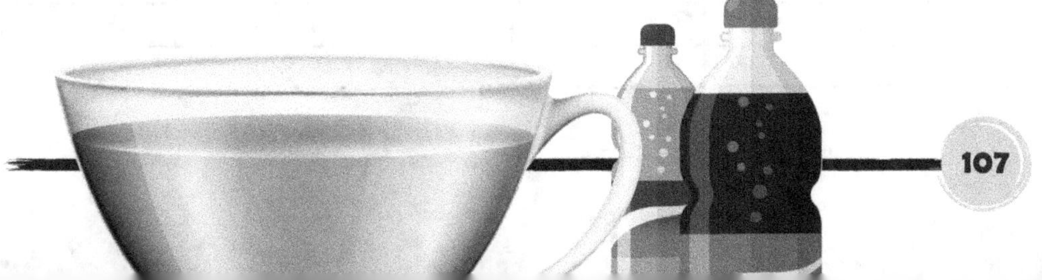

OTHER FOODS

FOOD for 100 g (3.5 Oz)	ENERGY Kcal	PROTEINS grams	CARBS grams	FATS grams
Mustard	80	5	6	4
Ketchup	110	1,5	25	0,5
Maple syrup	270	0	67	0
Agave syrup	305	0	76	0
Glucose syrup	310	0	78	0
Honey	320	0	80	0
Flour (wheat/corn)	350	10	73	2
Brown sugar	390	0	98	0
White sugar	400	0	99,8	0
Mayonnaise	690	1	3	75
Vegetable oil	900	0	0	100

CALORIE INTAKE PER DAY

BREAKFAST

FOOD	QUANTITY	ENERGY Kcal	PROTEINS grams	CARBS grams	FATS grams
TOTAL					

LUNCH

FOOD	QUANTITY	ENERGY Kcal	PROTEINS grams	CARBS grams	FATS grams
TOTAL					

COLLATION

FOOD	QUANTITY	ENERGY Kcal	PROTEINS grams	CARBS grams	FATS grams
TOTAL					

DINNER

FOOD	QUANTITY	ENERGY Kcal	PROTEINS grams	CARBS grams	FATS grams
TOTAL					

TOTAL FOR THE DAY

TARGET IN KCAL	INTAKE	DEFICIT

CALORIE INTAKE PER DAY

BREAKFAST

FOOD	QUANTITY	ENERGY Kcal	PROTEINS grams	CARBS grams	FATS grams
TOTAL					

LUNCH

FOOD	QUANTITY	ENERGY Kcal	PROTEINS grams	CARBS grams	FATS grams
TOTAL					

COLLATION

FOOD	QUANTITY	ENERGY Kcal	PROTEINS grams	CARBS grams	FATS grams
TOTAL					

DINNER

FOOD	QUANTITY	ENERGY Kcal	PROTEINS grams	CARBS grams	FATS grams
TOTAL					

TOTAL FOR THE DAY

TARGET IN KCAL	INTAKE	DEFICIT

* 9 7 9 8 3 2 0 1 2 5 1 5 2 *